Acknowledgements

The Association is grateful for the specialist help provided by the BMA committees and many outside experts and organisations, and would particularly like to thank Professor Jon Nicholl and Dr Wim Rogmans. In addition to the references and websites cited, we are most grateful for the assistance and information received from the following individuals: Lisa Cohen Barrios, Kathy Kaufer Christoffel, Arthur Kellermann, John Langley, Terry Nolan, Barry Pless, Fred Rivara and Alison Sewell.

Contents

1 Introduction   1

BMA policy on injury   1
Aims and scope of this report   4

2 Injuries: the scale of the problem and opportunities for prevention   7

Introduction   7
The burden due to injuries   8
    National and international comparisons   8
    Trends over time   9
    The burden on the poorest   10
    The impact of non-fatal injuries   10
    Long-term consequences   11
Causes of injury   12
    All ages   12
    Children   13
    Young people   13
    Older people   13
How can injuries be prevented?   14
    Prevention approaches   15
    Preventing unintentional injuries   17
    Children   18
    Child pedestrian injuries   19
    Young people   20
    Older people   20
    Intentional injuries   21
    Health inequalities and injury prevention   23
    From research into action   24

3 The economic burden of injury 27

Why should we invest in injury prevention? 27

Measuring the economic burden of injury 28

Relating burden of injury to the investment in injury
research and development 30
    The burden of injury and injury research and
    development investment in the UK 32
    Injury research 35
    Investment in injury prevention 36

Measuring the cost-effectiveness of injury prevention 36
    Quality Adjusted Life Years (QALY) 37
    Other measurement methods of cost-effectiveness 39

Implementation of effective injury prevention measures 40

The other potential benefits of injury prevention 43

4 Injury surveillance 45

Introduction 45

What is injury surveillance? 45

Characteristics of successful injury surveillance 47

Key issues 48
    Counting the occurrence of injury 49
    Exposure to risk 50
    Disablement resulting from improved survival 50

The building blocks — current UK national injury data
systems 51
    Underlying weaknesses in present UK injury data 51

Examples of UK local and regional injury surveillance 55
    PHISSCH, Newcastle 55
    CHIRPP, Glasgow 56
    AWISS, Wales 56

Other countries' national injury surveillance systems   56

International injury surveillance   58

5 Research & development in injury prevention   59

Current issues   59

Research process and infrastructure   60

Research funding   63

Research monitoring and information dissemination   66

6 Towards a national policy   69

Introduction   69

UK policy structures for injury prevention   70

Health policies   70

Transport and environmental policies   72

Fire, policing and crime prevention policies   74

Consumer affairs and consumer safety   76

Education and early years   76

Other government departments   77

Non-governmental bodies   78

The need for co-ordination   79

Recommendations   81

     Injury surveillance   81

     Research and development   83

     Implementation and strategic policy development   84

Appendix 1: International approaches to injury control 87

Introduction   87

International policy making   87

European Union   88

The United States of America   90
    Co-ordination of injury control at a national level in
    the United States of America   90
    State injury prevention co-ordination   90
    Surveillance   91
    Research   91
    Evaluation   92

Australia   92
    Co-ordination of injury control at a national level in
    Australia   92
    National surveillance of injury occurrence   93
    Approaches to the national co-ordination of research 93
    State and territorial links   94

New Zealand   94
    Co-ordination of injury control at a national level in
    New Zealand   94

Summary   95

References 97

Index 113

1

Introduction

The British Medical Association (BMA) is the professional organisation representing doctors in the UK. The Board of Science and Education was established to support the Association in its founding aim "to promote the medical and allied sciences and to maintain the honour and interests of the medical profession". Part of the remit of the Board is to undertake research studies on a wide range of key public health issues on behalf of the Association and to provide reports and guidance to the profession as well as information to the public on health related matters which are of general concern. When endorsed by BMA Council, the reports are published as BMA policy to inform and influence doctors, the NHS, government, policy-makers, the professions, the media and the public.

BMA policy on injury

The second edition of the BMA's policy report The BMA guide to living with risk,[1] published in 1990, presented a comprehensive review of the nature of risk and the major causes of death and injury that relate to occupation, transport, the home, natural disasters, etc. It also introduced new information on the risks to health in childhood caused by sudden infant death syndrome and unintentional injuries. To the extent that available data permitted, the report represented an attempt to put risk and injury into perspective and concluded that it is likely that advances in science including medical science will lead to longer lives, experienced at a generally higher level of well being. Many risks, such as the risk of injury, can be managed and reduced, but this is not true for all risks and none can be reduced to zero. It seemed important therefore that our increased capacity to identify, measure and control risks should be accompanied by a high level of public understanding of their significance. In order to reduce the risk of injury, education about the potential risks, particularly parental education, should be encouraged as a preventive measure.

November 1998 saw the launch at a BMA conference of Action on Injury[2] — a policy-makers' briefing document, setting the agenda for injury prevention amongst children and young people in the UK, prepared by a joint Royal Colleges working group. The report concluded that injury forms the single most common cause of death under the age of 40 years, is a major health burden for young people, and one of the four public health priority issues identified in Our Healthier Nation.[3]

The BMA policy report Growing up in Britain: Ensuring a healthy future for our children,[4] published in June 1999, provided a comprehensive overview on key aspects of child health including injury and abuse. The BMA commented that although the UK may be a member of the elite G8 group of leading industrial economies, its international ranking on key child health indicators is poor.

The BMA concluded:

- child injury is the greatest cause of childhood mortality and a considerable cause of morbidity after the first year of life.

- child injury deaths show the most pronounced social class gradient of any cause of death. Social class V has the highest rate.

- the majority of injuries to children under 5 occur in the home, and explanations for them centre around poverty and poor housing conditions.

- the UK has no single agency with responsibility for prevention of unintentional injury to children. The BMA recommended a national framework that would be the responsibility of government, health authorities and local authorities.

The complex issues surrounding risk from work activities and the many occupational environments are not considered in detail in this present report because of the wide ranging topics, policy areas and legislation that this would involve. The Royal Society summarised the average death rates at work in the UK.[5] Nearly twenty years later, the same pattern of risk to health is found overall but with a few significant changes: clothing manufacturing has become safer, with the lowest rate of accidental deaths at work, ie 5/million. Even deep-sea fishing (accidents at sea) has shown appreciable improvement, down from 2,800/million at risk in the 1970s, to 840/million for the period 1987-90. The Health and Safety Commission (HSC) and Executive (HSE) are now giving priority to industries with the highest accident rates. In addition to regulating the railways and Britain's major hazard industries, the HSC strategic plan prioritises eight key programmes of activity over the next three years. Three of the targets focus on specific industries — construction, agriculture, and the health service sector — where HSC considers there is a pressing need for health and safety improvements. Four programmes will prioritise specific issues: musculoskeletal disorders, work-related stress, workplace transport, and falls from heights. The eighth priority is to reduce slips, trips and falls within the local authority-enforced sector.[6] The BMA guide to living with risk and subsequent publications[7,8,9,10] have addressed some risks to health at work and particular injuries in detail, and the BMA continues to raise specific matters such as risks of injury in healthcare environments on a regular basis.

Aims and scope of this report

This publication presents new BMA policy on injury prevention, and focuses on people in all age groups and the burden of mortality and morbidity due to injuries from any cause.

For the purpose of the report, 'injury' is a broad term covering a multitude of types of health problems each of which have different factors associated with increased risk, and for which different types of interventions are possible. Intentional injuries include homicide and interpersonal violence, wars and other forms of collective violence, as well as suicide and other forms of self-harm. Unintentional injuries are typically classified according to the means of their occurrence: poisoning, burns and scalds, drowning, falls or transport-related.[11] The term 'accident' is avoided in the main, in keeping with international practice, as the extent of injuries goes well beyond those caused by accidents alone.

Chapter 2 provides an overview of the scale of the problem and trends of injury over time with both a national and international comparison. The personal factors relating to the individuals involved, environmental factors, socio-economic factors and lifestyle factors as well as other influences are discussed. Chapter 3 discusses the methods used internationally to measure the economic burden of injury and the national responses to this burden. It addresses the cost effectiveness of injury prevention in relation to the loss of potential healthy life years or disability adjusted life year measures for those affected.

Chapter 4 considers the need for systematic collection, analysis, interpretation and timely dissemination of health data for the planning, implementation and evaluation of public health programmes. The current UK national injury data systems and their weaknesses are discussed in detail. The specific problems associated with accidents or injuries caused by unintentional influences are considered in chapter 5. Particular reference is given to the need for improvements in the research infrastructure and the development of the academic aspects of injury prevention, together with the need for new approaches from the government and research funding organisations.

The concluding section (chapter 6) outlines current national structures responding to the problem of injury, and draws together the key aspects of injury prevention discussed within the report. It presents a broad range of recommendations for actions that need to be taken, primarily by government, both at Westminster and through devolution by the National Ministries in Scotland, Wales and Northern Ireland, in a co-ordinated and structured manner. The potential benefits that may arise from the possible diversity of approaches used in the devolved ministries should be utilised in order to ascertain the most effective methods of prevention policy.

This BMA policy report presents a comprehensive overview of the current challenges for government, in improving the surveillance and prevention of injury in the UK. It will be a valuable resource for doctors and all healthcare professionals working in the field of injury prevention, as well as those involved in health policy, transport and environmental issues, fire, policing and crime prevention, and education. These, together with many other specialities — will find this report a useful resource and a guide to supporting the need for an integrated system of surveillance and injury prevention in the UK. We hope this report will be a useful reference point for their on-going work.

2

Injuries: the scale of the problem and opportunities for prevention

Introduction

Injuries are a major cause of death and disability in the world today. The World Health Organization (WHO) has estimated that 5.8 million people world-wide died from injuries in 1998.[1] This figure is predicted to rise dramatically over the next two decades to 8.4 million in 2020.[2] Injuries are a 'disease', which kill nearly 20,000 UK citizens each year. Injuries require 30 million annual visits for medical attention,[3] waste twice as many pre-retirement life years as coronary heart disease, and consume at least 5% of health service expenditure.[4]

In the UK, injuries, whether unintentional or purposely inflicted, have been recognised as posing significant threats to the health of the population.[5,6,7,8] In England and Northern Ireland,[9] national targets have been set to reduce the burden due to injuries. The Information and Statistics Division of the NHS Common Services Agency is expected to produce national criteria for injury data collection for Scotland.[10] This chapter reviews what is known about the scale of the problem and who is at risk, and provides an introduction to the published literature on effective methods of injury prevention.

The burden due to injuries

World-wide almost 16,000 people die from injuries each day.[11] For every person that dies, several thousands more suffer non-fatal injuries, many of them suffering permanent disability. The greatest burden of injuries falls on the most vulnerable — the old and the young. Injury is the greatest threat to life in children and young people in the UK today, while older people are also at a greater risk of injury death. Each year in England and Wales, around 4,600 people aged 75 and over die as a result of injury, largely due to falls.

Furthermore, injuries are both caused by, and are a cause of, significant health inequalities. Injuries often result in massive health and lost productivity costs (see chapter 3). Injuries cause immense pain and suffering to victims and their families, with the burden on them and the services that treat and care for them being considerable.

National and international comparisons

Although the overall average annual mortality rates from injuries in the UK, particularly for children aged 1-14 years, compares favourably with EU countries, there is scope for considerable improvement. It has been estimated that if the UK could achieve the lowest European death rate for each injury type, child injury deaths (in the UK) could be reduced by 35-40%.[12]

Within the UK, there are considerable regional variations. Scotland and Northern Ireland show significantly higher rates of injury than in England and Wales, although some of these differences may be due to regional differences in the classification and recording of injury deaths.

Table 1: Injury deaths, age standardised rates per 100,000 population, both sexes (annual average over 5 year periods 1989-93 and 1994-98)[13,14,15]

	England & Wales		Scotland		Northern Ireland		Total UK	
	1989-1993	1994-1998	1989-1993	1994-1998	1989-1993	1994-1998	1989-1993	1994-1998
Unintentional injuries	18.1	16.4	28.2	26.2	26.2	24.8	19.8	14.9
	(10,900)	(10,453)	(1,697)	(1,444)	(435)	(408)	(13,033)	(12,304)
Homicide	0.6	0.6	2.4	2.1	5.4	4.3	0.9	0.8
	(324)	(329)	(128)	(105)	(84)	(68)	(537)	(502)
Suicide	7.2	6.4	10.6	11.6	8.3	8.8	7.6	7.0
	(3,834)	(3,498)	(554)	(618)	(127)	(126)	(4,516)	(4,242)
Undetermined intent	3.6	3.6	4.1	4.4	1.2	1.3	3.6	3.7
	(1,902)	(1,940)	(221)	(235)	(18)	(19)	(2,142)	(2,194)

Trends over time

Injury deaths in the UK have fallen by around 8% over the last decade. This decline is the result of a combination of factors including better trauma care, improvements in safety practice, and changing lifestyles. Greater reliance on the car and a reduction in the number of children and young people walking or cycling has reduced young people's risk of injury, but at the expense of decreased physical activity and freedom.[16]

The downward trend in unintentional injuries masks significant regional differences as well as differences between age groups and injury types. The greatest improvement has been made in child injury deaths while gains in other age groups have been more modest. The death rate due to homicide and self-inflicted injury has remained largely unchanged over the last decade.

The burden on the poorest

Although everyone is at risk of injury, the evidence is clear that the poorest in society are at far greater risk. As previously stated, injuries are both caused by, and are a cause of, significant health inequalities in the UK today. This gap between the richest and the poorest worsened during the 1980s and early 1990s.

Table 2: Trends in injury deaths in England and Wales by social class (rates per 100,000)[17,18]

	Children (age 0-15)				Adult men (age 20-64)			
	Unintentional injury		Intentional injury		Unintentional injury		Suicide and undetermined injury	
Social Class	1979-1983	1989-1992	1980-1983	1992-1995	1979-1983	1991-1993	1979-1983	1991-1993
I	24	16	0.3	0.3	17	13	16	13
II	25	16	0.4	0.4	20	13	15	14
IIIn	24	19	0.4	0.5	21	17	18	20
IIIm	36	34	0.7	0.8	27	24	16	21
IV	47	38	0.9	1.2	35	24	23	23
V	85	83	1.8	2.8	63	52	44	47

The impact of non-fatal injuries

Only a small proportion of the injuries that occur in the United Kingdom result in death, but the burden due to non-fatal injuries is considerable. Each year, some 720,000 people are admitted to hospital in England and Wales, in excess of 6 million visits[23] are made to accident and emergency departments, and one in seven people consult their GP for treatment of an injury.[24] The economic impact of injury is considered in more detail in chapter 3.

Figure 1: Pyramid of injury[19,20,21,22]

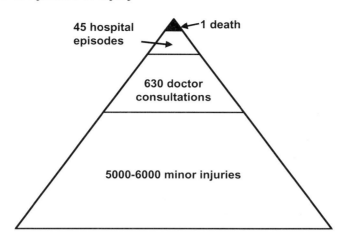

Long-term consequences

Many of those who survive the initial stages of injury go on to suffer long-term consequences. Injury-related disability can have a devastating effect on those affected. A study of the survivors of major trauma in one region of England showed that at five years post-injury, one in ten suffered severe disability and were dependent on carer support. Half of those of working age were not in paid employment.[25]

Injury also has less immediate consequences that can have a profound impact on those affected. For example, one in two of those who survive major trauma may suffer post-traumatic stress disorder.[26] The anticipation of injury can also be debilitating: fear of falling can lead to unnecessary limitation of activities and institutionalism in the elderly; while fear of violent crime can have a debilitating impact on individuals and local communities.[27]

Causes of injury

Many different factors influence people's risk of injury and the type of injury that occurs. These include personal factors relating to the individual or individuals involved, environmental factors, socio-economic factors and lifestyle factors. Some individuals have high-risk lifestyles through participating in dangerous sports that may result in potentially serious injuries if things going wrong. The magnitude of the risk taken could be reduced through encouraging people to learn about risk-taking, how to manage them, effective training, and the use of proper facilities and equipment. However, overall, only a small amount of injury is caused by risk behaviour.

Table 3: Risk factors for injury

Risk factor	Examples
Personal	Age, gender, ethnicity, physical and mental health, level of education about risk of injuries
Environmental	Home, work, leisure, transport, public places, eg poor lighting, unfenced swimming pool, lack of smoke alarm
Socio-economic	Poor quality over-crowded housing, unemployment
Lifestyle	Use of alcohol, drugs, smoking, risk-taking behaviour, eg speeding, no seatbelt

All ages

Road traffic accidents are a leading cause of death in most age groups. In 1998, almost 3,500 people were killed on UK roads with over 40,000 seriously injured.[28] Risk of road traffic injury varies by age and place of residence. For example, a serious accident on a rural road will on average involve 1.24 serious casualties compared with 1.08 serious casualties on an urban road, together with a greater amount of vehicle damage.[29]

Children

Although road traffic accidents are the leading cause of injury deaths throughout childhood, very young children are particularly vulnerable to injury within the home, including drowning, poisoning and fire. In 1998, 76 children under 5 years in England and Wales died as a result of an unintentional home injury, most commonly due to house fires, while some 700,000 were treated at accident and emergency departments.[30]

Older children are at greatest risk of death or injury on the roads. In 1998, 5,448 children aged under 15 years were killed or seriously injured on British roads. Of these, 3,737 were pedestrians, with a further 915 injured while cycling.[31] This figure is likely to be an underestimate as many injuries where no motor vehicle is involved are not reported to the police and consequently do not appear in the road statistics. Many of these children were killed or injured close to their own homes.[32]

Young people

In 1998, over half the deaths of young people aged 15-24 in England and Wales were due to injuries. Of these, two thirds were unintentional injury deaths, largely due to road traffic accidents. Of the intentional injury deaths, just under two thirds were self-inflicted.

Older people

In older age groups, falls are a major problem, with rates of falling in people aged 65 and over increasing exponentially with age.[33] Thirty percent of older people aged 65 and over fall each year, and this increases to 50% for people aged 80 and over. Seventy-five percent of fall-related deaths occur in the home. Deaths due to falls in people aged over 65 have increased over the last decade. Predicted increases in the number of elderly people in the UK mean that fall-related injuries such as hip fractures are expected to rise 2-3 fold over the next 25-40 years. For example, in a typical Primary Care Group population of 100,000 people, in an average year, 420 of those aged 50 and over are admitted to hospital due to a fall, a figure predicted to rise to 1,200 by 2030. Similarly, the number admitted to hospital with a hip fracture is expected to rise from 140 to 400 per 100,000 over the same period.[34]

How can injuries be prevented?

Injuries do not occur by chance. They are largely preventable, non-random events and not 'accidents'. Certain groups of people with certain characteristics are more likely to be injured — just as people who smoke are more likely to develop certain cancers and other diseases. Patterns of injury vary with a person's age, their gender, where they come from, where they live, and their lifestyle. By studying how injuries vary within the population, we can begin to gain an understanding of the factors that lead to injury and how the risk of injury may be reduced. Similar approaches to studying chronic disease has led to major advances in disease prevention.

Unlike many areas of illness prevention, effective measures of injury prevention can often achieve a very rapid reduction in mortality and morbidity if implemented fully. Yet, there is still much we do not know about injury cause and prevention effectiveness. Even where there is good evidence of intervention effectiveness, often safety measures are not being implemented and preventable injuries are still occurring. The health sector has an important role to play in all aspects of injury prevention, and systems of injury care should be imposed to prevent avoidable mortality and morbidity.

Prevention approaches

As with other areas of disease prevention, prevention of injuries may be primary, secondary or tertiary:

Tertiary prevention	The optimal treatment and rehabilitation of the injured person to minimise the impact of injury
Secondary prevention	The prevention or reduction of injury severity in incidents which do happen
Primary prevention	The prevention of circumstances which lead to injury

Tertiary prevention

Even with the advances that have been made in preventing the occurrence of injuries, we will never live in a risk-free world. The assumption that those who are injured always receive optimal care was first challenged in North America.[35] Case reviews in the UK confirmed that up to a third of trauma deaths are avoidable if appropriate systems of care are in place.[36] Over the last decade improvements in trauma services have made important contributions to the reduction in deaths, but there remains evidence of significant variation in UK hospital performance.[37,38] Data on the extent of avoidable disability are more difficult to obtain, but available evidence points to substantial unnecessary short and long-term suffering.[39]

In terms of rehabilitation medicine, (the active process that assists disabled people to acquire the knowledge and skills to maximise their own physical, psychological and social function), the demand for effective systems will increase as people live longer with substantial disability. A review of service provision in the UK found it to be insufficient or unavailable to many patients, with poor service for older people particularly.[40] In 2000 there were only 120 consultants and 40 specialist registrars working in the rehabilitation field, and the Royal College of Physicians recommended that the national objective should be one specialist in rehabilitation for every 250,000 of the UK population.[41] Research into the effectiveness and cost-effectiveness of rehabilitation interventions is also urgently required to ensure victims of injury receive the best possible chances of recovery.

With regards to head injury rehabilitation in particular, comparatively little attention and funding has been received.[42] This is despite increasing evidence of the efficacy of comprehensive multi-disciplinary rehabilitation compared to natural recovery from brain injury.[43] Extra resources and specialist staffing are necessary to expand the facilities in the UK to a level commensurate with the numbers of patients presenting with head injuries. Tertiary prevention thus continues to have an important role in the reduction of avoidable deaths and disability due to injury.

Primary and secondary prevention

The decline in the rate of deaths due to injury seen in the UK and other European countries over the last decades are, in part, a measure of the gains that have been made in injury prevention.

Table 4: Example for prevention of child unintentional poisoning[44]

	Individual	Injury-reducing agent	Environment
Pre-event	Child's developmental stage/parental behaviour	Use of child safety cap on medicine container	Availability of locked medicine cabinet
Event	Child's age	Dosage of medicine in container	Use of cabinet
Post-event	Parental knowledge of first aid	Labelling on medicine container	Access to and response of emergency services

Broadly, approaches to unintentional injury prevention can be divided into education (provision of information and training), environmental change (modification of products/environment, or use of additional safety devices), and enforcement (usually through regulation or legislation). The prevention of intentional injury is less easily categorised, relying not only on the above approaches, but also on community and family support, cognitive-behavioural interventions, and action aimed at reducing social exclusion.

Preventing unintentional injuries

The overall reduction in injury deaths seen in the UK in recent years is almost wholly due to reductions in the number of deaths due to unintentional injuries. There are many examples of effective injury prevention interventions that have contributed to a reduction in injury and death within the whole population or in selected high-risk groups. The most effective strategies tend to be those that adopt a combined approach where enforcement and/or environmental change have been backed up by an effective programme of education and training. Examples of the effectiveness of such an approach can be seen in many areas of life including transport and road safety, the workplace, safer building design and the leisure environment. Since the introduction of drink driving legislation and a systematic programme of public education over the last 15 years, fatal accidents involving alcohol have fallen 2.3% faster per year than fatalities generally, and serious accidents at a rate of 4.4% faster.[45]

Other interventions have been targeted at specific high-risk groups, eg children, young people and the elderly, reflecting the very different injury experience of different sections of the population. The need to prioritise these groups is also highlighted at a national level.[46,47,48]

Children

A range of changes to building legislation and product design have been introduced over the years in an attempt to make the home environment safer. For example, the introduction of regulations enforcing the compulsory use of child resistant safety containers for all children's aspirin and paracetamol preparations in 1976 led to a dramatic fall in the number of children admitted to hospital with unintentional poisoning as a result of these medications.[49] However, a clear relationship between such measures and reduced injuries is sometimes hard to establish.[50]

There is evidence that a combined approach where environmental change is backed up by enforcement and education can save lives. For example, the introduction of legislation in Washington State requiring new water heaters to be pre-set at a maximum 49°C combined with an educational campaign to inform people about the risks of excessively hot water led to a 56 % reduction in child admissions with tap water burns and scalds.[51] A further example is of a campaign in inner city New York that combined free window guards for those living in high rise buildings, together with a mass media campaign, home inspection, and local regulation for landlords. The campaign led to a 50% decrease in falls and a 35% decrease in child deaths.[52]

The effectiveness of smoke alarms in reducing death from house fire is well established. When a house fire occurs, one of the most important risk factors for death is the absence of a smoke alarm.[53] Smoke alarms are a reliable, inexpensive means of providing an early warning. In the USA, a give-away programme which distributed over 10,000 free smoke alarms to high risk homes in a deprived area of Oklahoma City led to an 80% reduction in fire related injuries in the target area.[54] Despite this, 20% of British households with children under 15 years do not have a smoke alarm.[55] A community give-away programme similar to that undertaken in Oklahoma has recently been successfully undertaken in the UK, although the effectiveness of this London-based programme is not yet known.[56]

Child pedestrian injuries

Although British children spend similar or less time out walking or cycling on roads than their European neighbours, their chances of being killed on the road are twice the European average. A recent study showed that approximately half of the difference in injury rates between the UK and The Netherlands and France could be explained by British children's greater exposure to busier main roads.[57] Transport policies which aim to regulate traffic flow in residential areas and separate traffic from pedestrians have been shown to have a significant impact on children's use of the environment and on injury rates.[58]

A scheme in The Netherlands that excluded most local traffic from residential areas and limited the speed of remaining traffic led to a 25% reduction in injuries. A similar scheme in five areas of the UK which redistributed local traffic and improved the safety of individual roads resulted in a 13% reduction in injuries.[59]

The introduction of 20mph speed limit zones in parts of the UK resulted in local reductions in child road accidents involving cyclists of 48% and a reduction of 70% in child road accidents involving pedestrians.[60]

Table 5: Speed kills[61]

Increasing speed leads to greater risk of child pedestrian death:	
At 20 mph	5% are killed
At 30 mph	45% are killed
At 40 mph	85% are killed

Young people

There have been relatively few injury prevention interventions reported which specifically target young people, although legislative measures to improve road and workplace safety in general have also led to reductions in injuries in this age group.[62] There is good evidence that the use of motorcycle and cycle helmets reduces injury risk. Legislation on motorcycle helmet use resulted in a reduction in motorcycle deaths. In the United States the repeal of motorcycle helmet use has been followed by an increase in fatalities of 25-40%.[63,64] A recent review of the evidence on the use of helmets by cyclists concluded that if correctly fitted, cycle helmets reduced the risk of head and brain injury by 63-88%.[65] In many sports, risk of injury has been reduced by rule changes or by use of protective devices.[66]

Older people

A number of interventions have been shown to be effective in reducing the risk of falls in older people. An example of a risk factor of falls is the medication that an individual may be taking.[67,68] The most successful falls prevention strategies use a multi-faceted approach involving both medical assessment of the individual and environmental assessment of where they live.[69] A London based study which adopted such a multi-faceted approach led to a 61% reduction in risk of falling, a 67% reduction in risk of recurrent falls and a 39% decrease in rate of hospital admission due to fall injuries.[70]

National evidence-based guidelines for fall prevention[71] emphasise the importance of:

• focusing on older people who are at greatest risk of falling

• assessment of these older people for their risk of a future fall focusing on the most important modifiable risk factors

- facilitating the modification of these risk factors either through direct intervention or through referral.

    Older people at greater risk of injury include:

- people who have recently fallen and consulted a health professional

- ambulant people living in an institutional setting

- people living in the community currently being visited by health and social care professionals

- people over 80.

Intentional injuries

Unlike unintentional injuries, the rate of death due to suicide and violence in the UK has shown little evidence of a decline. Prevention strategies for intentional injuries are relatively under-researched and, in general, are poorly understood. Suicide is a comparatively rare event making it difficult to mount large studies of an intervention's effectiveness. It is generally accepted that limiting the availability of methods of self-harm, for example by detoxification of domestic gas and car emissions, can lead to a reduction in the number of suicides.[72,73] People with mental health problems are at particular risk of suicide. The recently published National service framework for mental health services in England[74] outlines six standards for how local health and social care services can help to prevent suicide.

There is a similar dearth of evidence relating to the effectiveness of interventions intended to prevent violence and abuse. Deterrence and control of violence via the criminal justice system can reduce injury but does not impact on the underlying factors that lead to violent behaviour. There are promising signs that programmes of home visiting to families with young children can have a beneficial effect on rates of childhood injury, both unintentional and those from abuse.[75] Other potentially beneficial interventions include cognitive-behavioural approaches such as parenting skills programmes, anger control and family therapy.[76] Alcohol consumption shows a strong correlation with injury and violence. A review of interventions for preventing injuries in problem drinkers suggested that reducing alcohol consumption would lead to reductions in the rate of all injuries including suicide, domestic violence and assault.[77]

Intentional injury and violence can also occur in crowd situations. This may be explained to some extent by a process of deindividuation,[78] where aggression may result due to a reduction in the inhibition against anti-social behaviour when individuals are part of a group. This in turn may lead to a change in self-perception and perception of others, causing a loss of individuality and an increase in anonymity. Interventions to reduce the likelihood of aggressive behaviour have included the installation of CCTV allowing the identification of individual crowd members, police presence, and in the case of football crowds, the risk of being barred from travelling abroad and exclusion orders banning attendance of designated games.[79]

Unintentional injuries in crowds may occur due to the mismanagement of the venue. The Health and Safety Executive (HSE) commissioned research into crowd behaviour and highlighted physical risk factors that may result in over-crowding and possible injury:

- steep slopes

- dead ends, locked gates

- convergence of several routes into one

- uneven or slippery flooring/steps

- reverse or cross flows in a dense crowd

- flows which are obstructed by queues or gathering crowds

- large pedestrian flows mixing with animals or traffic

- moving attractions in a crowd.

As a result the HSE has produced guidance on managing crowds safely, detailing preventive action that may be taken by organisers.[80]

Health inequalities and injury prevention

There have been relatively few injury prevention initiatives that have been designed to meet the needs of the most deprived communities. In 1996, a review of the literature relating to the prevention of injuries in children identified 142 studies.[81] Of these, only 11 studies specifically mentioned that they were targeted at areas of deprivation and only one of these was from the UK.[82] The authors of this study, which was a home safety programme designed to encourage parents to reduce the presence of hazards in their home via mass media information and targeted home visits, emphasised the importance of tailoring safety education to the needs of disadvantaged families.

General safety campaigns that target the whole population may be preferentially taken up by people from more affluent areas, thus worsening the health divide. The recent smoke alarm give-away programme in Camden and Islington, mentioned previously, demonstrated that the most deprived households, where children are 15 times more likely to die in a house fire, can be successfully targeted.[83]

Measures to reduce the excess burden of injuries falling on the poorest in society have also been reviewed by the Independent inquiry into inequalities in health (The Acheson Report).[84] This report highlighted the strong link between injury and poverty, and social exclusion. The report makes a number of recommendations for reducing injury related health inequalities including action on unemployment, social exclusion, housing, transport and on lifestyle factors such as smoking and alcohol.

From research into action

Evidence of the effectiveness of an injury prevention intervention is of little value if that intervention is not implemented. Too often it can be many years between the development of an effective method of injury prevention and its widespread adoption into routine practice. For example, evidence of the effectiveness of car seat belts can be identified at least as early as 1967.[85] Health promotion campaigns were ineffective until the introduction of legislation enforcing the use of front seat belts in 1983 — some 17 years later. It is estimated that some 7,000 fatal or serious injuries were prevented in the first year following legislation.[86] The number of deaths or serious injuries that could have been prevented in the intervening years is unknown.

Still today, effective interventions are not being put into practice. Not all homes in the UK have a functioning smoke alarm, and perhaps an education programme informing people about checking their batteries could be considered. In addition, many toxic substances are dispensed in containers that are not child safe, and many old people are at risk from falling through easily remediable risk factors.

The implementation of injury prevention intervention requires action at a national, local and individual level. The national health strategy for England (Saving lives: Our healthier nation)[87] outlines a range of actions that individuals, local partnerships and national government can take, for example:

Action	Examples
Individual	Install and maintain smoke alarms
	Avoid drink driving
	Improve driving behaviour
Local partnerships	Increase smoke alarm ownership
	Introduce area-wide road safety measures
	Develop local safe routes to school
National	Promote fire safety
	Review housing fitness standards
	Co-ordinate government strategy

Other national initiatives such as the National service frameworks for older people[88] and Mental health[89] and national evidence-based guidelines should also lead to better implementation of effective injury prevention interventions. Health Action Zones[90] and healthy living centres[91] also offer the potential to target those more deprived areas at greater risk of injury.

Although it is clear that efforts to prevent injuries require action by a variety of organisations, the health sector has an important role to play in all aspects of injury prevention by:

- systematic collection of high quality data on injuries

- surveillance of injury trends and identification of high risk locations, groups, individuals or emerging injury risks

- working as part of a multi-disciplinary team to identify those at risk, and modify risk factors where appropriate

- providing optimal care and rehabilitation for those who are injured

- support and monitor national and local action to implement effective injury prevention interventions

- ensuring new interventions are rigorously evaluated

- via Primary Care Groups/local health groups, Health Authorities/Boards, and NHS Trusts, supporting other local agencies in ensuring that injury prevention is a priority area for action in local Health Improvement Programmes.

3

The economic burden of injury

The general burden of injury has been discussed in chapter 2. This chapter will concentrate specifically on the economic burden.

Why should we invest in injury prevention?

When a 'disease' such as injury primarily kills fit, young people, or may leave them incapacitated for life, then we should be investing heavily to understand its origins. When the value the public attach to avoiding injury exceeds thirty billion pounds annually,[1] then it is extraordinary that so little is invested in research to find a cure, or that known effective forms of prevention are not being fully implemented.

This chapter discusses the methods used internationally to measure the burden of injury and the national responses to this burden. It is difficult to make similar measurements in the UK due to deficiencies in the available information, therefore we review the nearest equivalent data for the UK. This burden is compared to that imposed by other national public health priorities (ie cancer and vascular disease). Relative investment in research and development is set alongside these disease burdens. To assess the potential return from greater involvement in injury prevention, the UK is compared to other developed countries for the extent to which known cost-effective preventive measures have been implemented and for evidence that lower injury rates are achievable.

Measuring the economic burden of injury

The national burden of injury can be described in a number of ways:

- Potential Years of Life Lost (PYLL) indicates the burden from fatalities due to injuries. PYLLs are calculated by subtracting age at death for fatalities, from normal life expectancy (conventionally 75 years in UK estimates). For example, 10 people dying at age 45 generate 300 PYLLs (that is, 30 unlived years each before age 75).

- disability Adjusted Life Years (DALY) indicate the burden from fatalities and disabilities due to injury. DALYs are made up of Potential Years of Life Lost (see PYLL definition) plus Years of Life Disabled (YLD) amongst those who survive with disability. YLDs indicate the number of healthy years lost through disability. For example, 10 further people who are 50% disabled since the age of 45 generate 150 further YLDs (50% × 300 PYLLs) which, when added to the 300 PYLLs above, creates 450 DALYs amongst 20 injured people.

- the direct costs of providing health and other services to those with injuries.

- the additional indirect costs to society of lost productive capacity.

- the much larger value which people place on avoiding the pain and suffering associated with injury.

Such wide ranging burden of injury accounts have been completed for the United States,[2,3,4,5,6,7] Canada,[8] Australia,[9] New Zealand,[10] and The Netherlands.[11] In the UK, such an analysis is confined to estimates of the direct costs[12] and to some more detailed valuations applied to injuries on roads and in the home.[13,14]

These studies reveal the huge costs attributable to injury in every developed country where this account has been calculated. In the USA the direct costs of treating injury are estimated at 12% of all US medical spending and amount to US$330 for every US citizen.[15] In the UK the direct costs exceed £1.6 billion annually[16] and when the amount the public express themselves 'willing to pay' to avoid injuries is included, the cost burden is at least twenty times greater.[17] In terms of the cost of childhood injury, it has been estimated that the value to society of prevention of injury in the home is £9,460 million.[18,19] There is no published UK account of indirect costs of injury (eg loss of earnings and dependency costs), but it is likely that this figure could approach £9 billion per annum.

Comparisons between countries of the economic burden are extremely sensitive to the costing and valuation methods used. There is also evidence that 'cost per injury case' (ie health spending, lost productivity) is directly related to the Gross National Product per capita of the countries concerned.[20]

More useful comparisons can be made within countries (or groups of countries), as in the World Health Organization (WHO) The global burden of disease study,[21] of the relative contribution of injury versus other public health problems. The WHO placed injury amongst the top 15 causes of Disability Adjusted Life Years (DALYs) lost at every age group under 60 years for 'European region high income countries' in 1998,[22] with the projection that the burden from injuries will increase globally by 2020 to a level exceeding infectious diseases. In the UK, attempts to measure the relative burden attributable to different diseases using DALYs are confined to small scale exercises with injury largely excluded for lack of appropriate data.[23] Comparisons including injuries have been made in the US, versus a variety of other conditions;[24,25] in Canada, versus HIV;[26] in Australia, versus other International Classification of Diseases ICD9 chapter based health care costs;[27] and in The Netherlands, versus six large disease-based categories.[28] These studies reveal the immense and increasing relative importance of injury as a public health problem across all developed economies.

Relating burden of injury to the investment in injury research and development

The literature on the relationship between the burden of injury and the investment in injury research and development is sparse and stems mostly from the United States. Thus, Injury in America in 1985[29] compared research investment to the numbers of Potential Years Life Lost from injury, cancer, heart disease and stroke.

In 1989, in a report to the US Congress, Rice et al[30] demonstrated that although injury caused more than twice the number of lost life years, the federal research expenditure on injury still lagged behind cancer or cardiovascular disease. These US comparisons have now been updated again for 1995 (figure 2[31]) and despite major investment in injury research, the relative picture is still largely the same.

These efforts in the United States to increase the political and scientific commitment to injury as a public health problem resulted in the establishment of the Centre for Injury Prevention and Control in Atlanta, which now has funding of US$70 million per annum, and which has in turn fostered the development of ten multi-disciplinary injury prevention and control research and development centres in universities across the United States. Similarly, in Australia, the publication of Looking forward to better

Figure 2: Potential Years of Life Lost (PYLL)* annually and federal research expenditure for major causes of death in the United States[32,33,34,35]

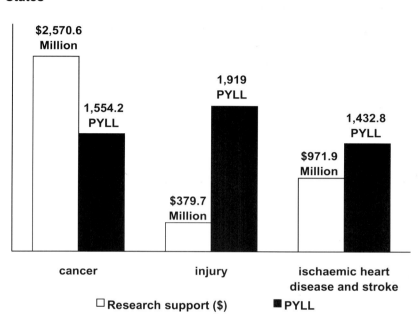

*Age adjusted years of potential life lost (PYLL) before age 75 in 1996 was calculated per 100,000 population. Injury included unintentional injury, homicide, and suicide. The research support for injury is for financial year 1995; research support for cancer, heart diseases, and stroke is NIH support for financial year 1996.

health[36] led to a strategic decision in 1998 to direct 18% of the Commonwealth Government's 'Better Health' funding to injury. This decision was followed by a widespread expansion of academic and service activity. New Zealand followed a similar pattern, starting with a New Zealand Medical Research Council (NZMRC) symposium in 1979 and leading to major multi-disciplinary research centres in Otago and Auckland.[37]

The WHO attempted to assess the relative spending on health research by condition across the world and their conclusion respecting injury is as follows:

"only limited information has been available ... [which] confirms [the] degree of neglect of this major cause of disease burden (anticipated 20% of all DALYs by 2020)"

In the same report, it is notable that the estimated public investment in all types of health research and development in the UK at 0.06% of GNP was towards the bottom of the EC league (only Greece and Spain were below) and was less than one third of that seen in Denmark, Austria or the USA.[38]

The burden of injury and injury research and development investment in the UK

In figures 3-5 we illustrate the situation in England and Wales, using a similar approach to that used for the US.

Figure 3a shows equivalent data for Potential Years of Life Lost (PYLL) in the UK due to cancer, injury and vascular disease as incorporated in figure 2 for the USA. When expressed as Potential Years of Life Lost for each death (figure 3b), then it is clear that the prevention of each injury death saves about three times more life years than preventing one cancer or vascular death, because the average age of injury is lower than that for cancer or heart disease and stroke.

Adjustment of these figures to take account of the extra years of healthy life lost by disabled survivors (ie to create DALYs by adding Years of Life Disabled to Potential Years of Life Lost) is difficult. There is little doubt that disability following injury is common, but there are no satisfactory data from which to create national DALY estimates in the UK. However, the pattern of relative DALY burden by disease group has been documented by the WHO for 'Established Market Economies'[40] and is likely to represent the situation in the UK. Figure 4 shows that the total burden in terms of overall potential healthy life years lost (ie DALYs) before age 75 approaches that for ischaemic heart disease and stroke combined. In Figure 5 it can be seen that when the

Figure 3: Burden of mortality in terms of Life Years Lost by cause, UK 1996-98[39]

Figure 3a: Potential Years of Life Lost (PYLL)

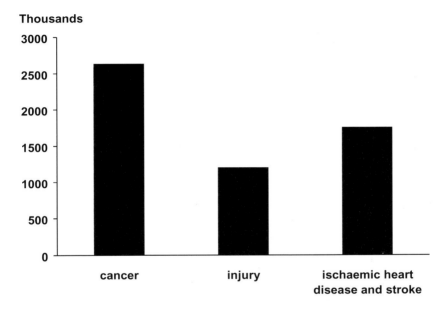

Figure 3b: Years of Life Lost per death

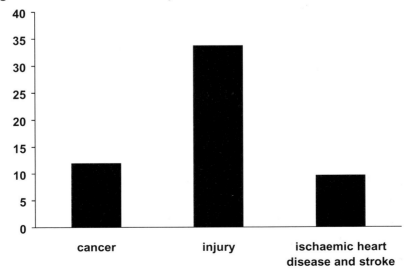

Figure 4: Disability Adjusted Life Years* lost by cause, UK 1996-98

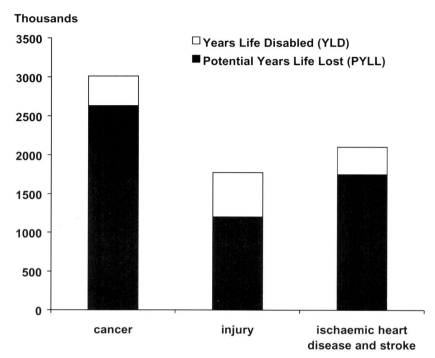

Thousands

Legend:
- □ Years Life Disabled (YLD)
- ■ Potential Years Life Lost (PYLL)

*YLL <75 and PYLL as for figure 3. YLD estimated at the same cause specific ratio to YLL as for Established Market Economies in WHO's *The global burden of disease*.[41] This greatly simplifies the WHO DALY method. Specifically, age weighting and discounting are not used and may be ethically questionable.[42]

proportion of DALYs in figure 4 attributed to living with disability (ie YLD) is examined separately, it is considerably higher for injury. Furthermore, these years of healthy life lost to disability are primarily people of working age.

Figure 5: Years Life Disabled by cause: UK 1996-98

Thousands

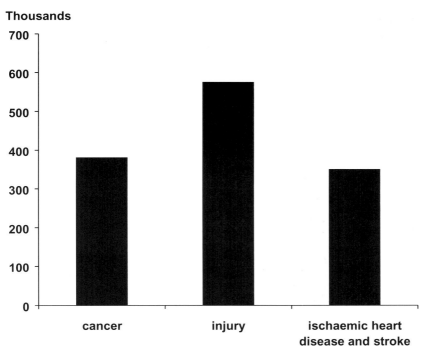

Injury research

The amount of research conducted into injury prevention is very small in comparison to its national burden (shown in figure 4). For example, the Medical Research Council spend on cancer research (1998-99) was £28.5 million, and £18.1 million on heart disease research (1999-2000). Spend on research into the prevention of accidental injuries was only £59,100 (1999-2000).[43] Charitable research investment in cancer and heart disease research is likely to be significant, while voluntary sector support for injury research is not likely to exceed £1.5m.

Investment in injury prevention

The amounts invested in injury prevention strategies are rarely accounted for. In the UK, the Parliamentary Advisory Committee on Transport Safety reported that while road deaths and injuries cost the nation £10.9 billion:

> "Combined Government spending on police enforcement, safety engineering, driver licensing and education total only £470 million."

This was contrasted with the massive increase in spending on rail safety following the Paddington rail crash, even though about 300 Britons die on the road for every rail death.[44]

The justification for spending on one form of prevention rather than another, whether based on types of injury or in comparison with other preventable public health problems, is of course contingent on knowledge of what prevention is effective and how much it costs to implement per avoided event. People may also prefer to spend more to avoid injury events over which they have little control.

This notion of the cost-effectiveness of interventions also needs to be complemented by information on the extent to which known effective interventions have been implemented (ie the net potential return from further investment in prevention). It has been argued that this measure is preferable to the use of disease burden to decide investment priority.[45,46] The approach might equally be used to consider the potential for a return from investment in research.

Measuring the cost-effectiveness of injury prevention

Injury prevention is not cheap. Indeed a characteristic of the passive safety provided by effective engineering of the physical environment, vehicles, and consumer products is the relatively high cost of universal protection. Similarly, enforcement of important safety legislation requires expensive training, monitoring and prosecutions to maintain effect. Those educational interventions which work to alter risky behaviour or to induce a wider culture of safety, and thereby prevent injuries, require substantial and constantly reinforced investment. It is important to ensure, therefore, not only that injury prevention works, but also that the benefits of avoided injury are achieved at an affordable cost.

A major benefit of injury prevention is avoided death. Because so much injury mortality is amongst young people, the savings in Potential Years of Lost Life for each avoided injury death are large. To this benefit should be added the avoided pain, suffering and continuing disability associated with simultaneous prevention of non-fatal injuries (figure 4). One method of estimating this benefit is to translate years of avoided injury disability and death into an equivalent number of Quality Adjusted Life Years (QALY) gained from injury prevention.

Quality Adjusted Life Years (QALY)

In the calculation of the QALY gain from an intervention, additional years of life are weighted by a value between 0 and 1 to reflect the quality of life in which they are spent.[47] A variety of methods have been developed by health economists to arrive at these weightings. The most common approach is where samples of the population are asked to state to what extent they prefer a range of different states of health described to them. The methods used include visual analogue methods, time trade-off methods and standard gamble methods.[48]

Calculating the estimated health gains from an intervention can be carried out very simply. If intervention A increases a patient's life expectancy, on average, by 5 years, and these 5 years are spent in perfect health (1.0), then the QALY gains from treatment A are calculated by multiplying the number of additional years of life gained by a weight which appropriately reflects the quality of life in which these additional years are spent. In this example, 5 QALYs are generated (1.0 × 5 = 5). If intervention B increases a patient's life expectancy by 5 years and these 5 years are spent in less than perfect health (0.6) then the QALY gains from intervention B are 3 QALYs (0.6 × 5 = 3).

The total number of QALYs gained from avoided death and disability is then set against the net cost of the preventive intervention to give a cost per QALY. Table 6 shows a set of such estimates developed in the US for childhood injuries. Where the savings exceed the costs, the cost per QALY saved is 0. The idea is that resources should be invested in health care interventions which produce QALYs at low cost.[49]

Table 6: Costs per QALY for selected injury prevention measures* (in 1997 US Dollars) [50]

Injury prevention measure	Cost per QALY
Child safety seat	<$0**
Zero tolerance of alcohol, drivers under age 21	<$0
Provisional licensing, midnight curfew	<$0
Bicycle helmet, ages 5-15	<$0**
Smoke detector	<$0
Childproof cigarette lighter	$4,000
Poison control centre	<$0

*All estimates were computed at a 3% discount rate and are compared with the absence of the intervention. The cost per QALY saved was computed by dividing the QALYs saved per unit by the net cost of the unit (which equals the unit cost minus the reduced medical care, property damage, insurance claims administration, and other direct costs). When these direct cost savings exceeded the cost of the safety measure, the cost per QALY saved is <$0.

** Ignores discomfort and inconvenience costs.

It will be seen that in many cases the cost of injury prevention is entirely paid for by the avoided treatment and property damage costs. Even if these savings in direct costs could not be realised or transferred to pay for prevention, the cost per QALY would still be very small compared to those associated with other generally implemented medical interventions, eg neonatal intensive care for babies between 1 and 1.5 kg ($10,000 per QALY).[51]

Further cost-effectiveness estimates for injury prevention initiatives at all ages are given by Miller and Levy[52] (80 examples) and Tengs et al[53] (131 examples). Of these, about one third show costs per QALY of less than $10,000.

Other measurement methods of cost-effectiveness

In the UK road safety field, a rather different method of economic analysis is used, in which the benefits of lives saved and avoided injuries are assigned a monetary value. This 'tariff', derived from surveys of public willingness to pay for reductions in risk, places a value of £1,207,670 on the avoidance of a death and £141,490 and £13,940 for avoidance of a single serious or slight injury respectively (1998 prices).[54] Using such figures, the benefit of the Urban Safety Programme (which demonstrated that residential traffic calming led to a 13% reduction in road casualties) was estimated to exceed the implementation costs within five years.[55] Similar analyses are used to justify engineering measures on major UK roads, such as motorway lighting.

Perhaps the most cogent demonstration of 'value for money' from injury prevention is where these savings are sufficient to drive commercial investment. In Victoria, Australia, the Traffic Accident Commission (providers of compulsory third party motor insurance for three million State residents) invests A$30 million annually in road safety programmes. In return, they estimate that reductions in road traffic accidents save A$100 million annually on their out-goings in victim compensation payments. If tariff values such as those above were used instead, then the returns would be A$300 million each year (ie ten times the amount invested).[56]

This demonstration of cost-effectiveness in injury prevention in Victoria covered a variety of interventions, from traditional road 'black spot' engineering, through to multi-faceted campaigns to control injuries from drink-driving, excessive speed and driver fatigue-related injuries. A vital component of the programme is support for Monash University Accident Research Centre in Melbourne. This multi-disciplinary academic unit provides analysis of local injury causes, informs programme design, and conducts evaluations of the outcomes from interventions. The cost-effectiveness of such research investment is hard to quantify, nevertheless the WHO, through its global forum for health research, has estimated that the potential gain in Disability Adjusted Life Years per research dollar should make injury research a high priority.[57]

Implementation of effective injury prevention measures

The penetration of proven (cost) effective measures to prevent injuries within the UK is not generally known. From the perspective of the population most at risk of injury, namely the young and the elderly, especially those in socially deprived environments, the extent of exposure to avoidable hazards is not monitored. This exposure could be as unprotected drivers/passengers in motor vehicles, as pedestrians in proximity to rapid traffic, as cyclists without adequately fitting cycle helmets, in playgrounds with poor surfacing and high fall risks, in houses without a functioning smoke alarm, or exposure to insecurely contained poisonous medications/household products — all preventable dangers.

It is important to estimate the extent of this unmet need for investment in prevention. The marginal cost of further increases in safety may, in some circumstances, be very high (eg air/train passengers, workplace fire protection) while some highly effective measures may be of lesser relevance within the UK setting (for example the fencing of domestic swimming pools). Priority should be given to those cost-effective interventions which address highly prevalent risks in the UK, and which are still not fully implemented. Evidence should also be established for the effectiveness of widely implemented injury prevention programmes for which, as yet, there is no evidence of effect.

Some indication of the priorities for injury prevention implementation within the UK can be deduced from the international literature. For instance, a comparison of child injury mortality across European countries suggests that if the best cause specific mortality rates from other EU countries were achieved in the UK, our child injury deaths could be cut by 40%.[58] The major contributors to this relative UK excess are household fire deaths in childhood, where UK rates are three and a half times those in Austria; child poisoning fatalities, where UK rates are more than five times those in Sweden; and, more important numerically, passenger road traffic accident deaths, which could be cut by one third if Danish rates were achieved. The most striking UK deficiency, however, is in pedestrian road traffic accidents, where UK child mortality is twice that in The Netherlands (and nearly four times that in Sweden).

Further exploration of this disparity in pedestrian risk between Dutch and English children has shown that this is not due to English children spending more time exposed to the road environment.[59] On the contrary, Dutch children are equally exposed; what differs is that in The Netherlands half of all child pedestrian time is spent in traffic calmed/speed controlled areas. In the UK only 10% of children are so protected.

With respect to child passenger protection in cars, the UK has a better record. However, observational studies in 1995 suggested that nearly 50% of UK child car passengers still travel either completely unrestrained or using inappropriate or incorrectly applied restraints.[60] A publication by the Organisation for Economic Co-operation and Development (OECD) revealed that other developed countries with similar legislation, such as Norway, Germany and Australia are much further advanced in the degree to which this protection of children is fully enforced.[61]

In the same OECD report, it is clear that the UK legislation for domestic fire protection is also relatively weak. Over the last ten years, Norway, Sweden and Ireland have introduced laws to require smoke detectors in all homes. State legislation is also in place in the USA, Canada and Australia for the same purpose.[62] Meanwhile, within the UK, the voluntary use of smoke alarms in homes, although apparently widespread, is specifically deficient in those households most at risk (socially deprived households with high prevalence of cigarette smokers), often due to the removal of batteries.[63] UK legislation is also weak with respect to domestic fire prevention. Smokers' materials cause more than a third of fatal house fires in the UK, yet there is no requirement in this country for cigarette lighters to be made child resistant. Such regulations have existed throughout the USA, Canada and Australasia for some years.[64] Recent legislative efforts in the USA and New Zealand are now directed towards the introduction of a mandatory standard for fire safe cigarettes.[65]

It might reasonably be concluded that there is potential within the UK to implement known cost-effective measures to prevent injury. Many effective interventions have not been subject to cost-effectiveness studies, for example, elderly fall 'clinics' and window bars, and little is known of the extent of their implementation. Furthermore, economic appraisals of transport, smoking and alcohol policies rarely consider injury frequency as a potential outcome, though changes in these risk factors could have profoundly beneficial effects in terms of injury reduction.

The other potential benefits of injury prevention

Changes in risks may lead to changes in behaviour. The potential for this is illustrated by international studies of children in traffic. Whereas only a quarter of Australian children aged 6-9 spend more than 15 minutes walking each day,[66] in Umea, Sweden, with safer roads, twice as many children this age achieve this degree of exposure to the road environment. Three times as many Australian children are taken to school by car, in contrast to Swedish children who are five times more likely to cycle to school by themselves.

A substantial part of the explanation for recent changes in UK child pedestrian mortality rates is a decrease in children's exposure to roads, as well as variations in traffic volume.[67] If pedestrian safety were improved through traffic calming, speed reductions and changes in traffic mix volume (eg from greater use of public transport) then there might be considerable health benefits for children from increased pedestrian access to the outside environment for play, school, travel etc (and economic benefits for parents, no longer required to supervise them).[68] At the moment the situation in the UK is so bad that 10% of children are never allowed outside to play because there is nowhere safe for them.[69] A similar argument might be applied to improving cycling safety, with even more direct health benefits, as well as the indirect advantages of reduced air pollution, noise, and wasted time in traffic jams.[70] Improved public transport and pedestrian safety will also benefit the vulnerable elderly, who are at high risk on urban roads, but who rely on outdoor access for exercise and social contact. This potential expansion of pedestrian and cycling access will of necessity produce some dis-benefits to others (for example, longer travel times, costs of public transport and road engineering).

Reductions in exposure to other injury risks may challenge powerful vested interests. Gun control is the obvious solution to the huge problem of firearm injury and death in the USA. To a lesser degree, a similar problem exists in Northern Ireland and increasingly in several UK cities. This has been partially addressed by gun legislation following the massacres at Hungerford and Dunblane, but much remains to be done. Injury reduction must also be counted amongst the health benefits of smoking and alcohol control. Fifteen percent of fatal road traffic accidents are associated with excess alcohol,[71] while over a third of house fires are ignited with tobacco smoking materials.[72]

4

Injury surveillance

Introduction

There is a widely quoted maxim in medicine that diagnosis should, as far as possible, precede treatment. In the public health setting, where the population is the patient, an analogous principle applies: that a community diagnosis is required before a public health intervention is implemented. For the purposes of injury prevention, two important pieces of information are necessary for community diagnosis. First, what is the epidemiology (frequency and nature) of injury in the population. And second, what are the main causes of injury that are amenable to intervention. This information comes from injury surveillance.

What is injury surveillance?

Surveillance is a population-based activity with a specifically public health function. Health surveillance has been defined as "the systematic collection, analysis, interpretation and timely dissemination of health data for the planning, implementation and evaluation of public health programmes".[1] The absence or inadequacy of data is a serious impediment to all public health efforts. By generating relevant data, surveillance should therefore facilitate prevention. On the other hand, data alone, however comprehensive, are only the starting point. Surveillance is a necessary first step, but is insufficient in itself unless linked to the epidemiological and public health literature on cause and effectiveness, and eventually to specific public health measures.

Data on injuries may be derived from a variety of sources within and outside the healthcare system. Some of the healthcare sources are routinely collected for administrative reasons and cover mortality, hospitalisations and visits to primary care clinics. Others are specially designed to generate epidemiological and aetiological information about injury. These so-called 'injury surveillance systems' instead are increasingly being developed throughout the world to meet the information needs of public health practitioners and other professionals with a remit for injury prevention. Injury surveillance systems commonly collect information not only about injury frequency, but also about the place of occurrence, circumstances, mechanism, products (if any) involved, nature of the injury, body part affected and possibly clinical activity. The latter is important if the potential benefits of tertiary prevention are to be realised. However, in general, the emphasis has been on the sequence of events leading to the injury rather than on information about clinical presentation, management and outcome. The success of injury surveillance systems is variable and few meet all of the quality criteria defined by specialist groups.[2]

Detailed epidemiological information about injury is required at local, regional, national and international levels. Locally and regionally, such information is useful for planning healthcare services, for developing and implementing safety policies, practices, standards and regulations, and for evaluating the effectiveness of preventive interventions. Nationally and internationally, injury information is important for policy making and priority setting by governments or trans-national agencies, for researchers investigating aetiology, epidemiology, treatment, outcome or prevention, and for a range of non-governmental, commercial and voluntary organisations with an interest in, or remit for, injury or safety.

Characteristics of successful injury surveillance

There is little methodological consistency in the different approaches to injury surveillance which have proliferated throughout the world. Data collection, coding and classification methods vary enormously as do sampling techniques. Some systems cover the whole population while others are restricted to specific age groups such as children or older people. Some collect information on specific types of injury while others are all-embracing. Although the majority identify injuries using clinical or administrative records, a few systems ascertain relevant events by population surveys. This heterogeneity creates virtually insurmountable difficulties in comparing the results across systems and has led to a number of recent initiatives designed to introduce a degree of standardisation of surveillance methods.

Total uniformity of injury surveillance methods may be neither desirable nor achievable. A consensus is emerging, however, that a number of key conditions should be met if an injury surveillance system is to achieve its full potential. These may be expressed as quality criteria,[3,4] including practicality, relevance, accessibility, validity, stability and effectiveness. Thus injury surveillance systems will require dedicated resourcing to avoid unrealistic burdens on front line staff and must demonstrate that they meet the needs of data users with complete, accurate and longitudinally stable information delivered at the required time and place.

Effectiveness

Case studies suggest that surveillance has made a significant impact on injury prevention policies and outcomes. For example, national surveillance of the causes of unintentional injury in the UK identified falls amongst older people as a priority area. This was subsequently embodied in a national policy document — Saving lives: Our healthier nation.[5] The Department of Trade and Industry commissioned a review of the patterns and trends in occurrence of falls linked to evidence of effectiveness of preventive interventions. Meanwhile, the Department of Health commissioned the development of guidelines for falls prevention. This work has been very influential in guiding the development of local Health Improvement Programmes for the prevention of falls amongst older people.

Road and vehicle engineers have for many years based design solutions for improved highway safety on analysis of long running injury surveillance systems for traffic accidents. A notable example is the mechanism of action and refinements in the design of airbags.[6] Similarly, the introduction of several successful consumer product regulations, such as Child Resistant Closures to prevent child aspirin poisoning, can be traced to effective use of injury surveillance data. Despite these, and other positive examples, limitations of the data systems that lie at the heart of UK-based surveillance systems hamper their effectiveness.

Key issues

Key outputs from injury surveillance include the rates of occurrence of injury and also their longer term consequences, by person, place, time and circumstance of injury. In order to measure a rate of injury, both the occurrence of the injury within the target population and the size of the population at risk need to be accurately measured. To represent the consequences of injury requires information on not only who dies but also the level of disablement, including loss of quality of life following the injury for those who survive their injury. The accurate measurement of each of these has its problems, as discussed in chapter 3.

Counting the occurrence of injury

In order to count the occurrence of any event/outcome, a clear definition of what is being counted is needed. The term 'injury' covers a wide range of injury types and severities, ranging from a scratch or bruise that is self-treated, to a skull fracture with brain injury that either results in death or permanent incapacity. It is impossible to envisage a system that would count all of these injuries, and so a clear definition of a case is necessary. In epidemiology, definitions are based on diagnosis, defects, pathology etc[7] since these are relatively stable and objective. In injury surveillance, as in other fields, the definition of injury should also take account of the severity of injury, and a case should be counted only if it exceeds a given severity threshold.[8]

All of the important current sources of UK data on non-fatal injury are based on a vague definition of an injury. These include:

- hospital admissions and attendance at an accident and emergency department (which are utilisation measures)

- police road traffic accident reports

- work accidents notified to the Health and Safety Executive (HSE), and

- fire statistics collected by fire services (which are reliant on reports from victims or others).

It is known that the use of hospital services depends on many factors including the supply of and access to the service, professional decision making, and the behaviour of various population groups. Consequently definitions based on utilisation of hospital services alone will result in biased and misleading information.[9] Similarly, reporting to the police, the fire service and the HSE is incomplete and varies across population groups, and so a definition of injury based on reporting to each of these systems will likewise result in biased and misleading information.

As a result of such uncertainties, it has been stated that we do not even know whether the rates of non-fatal injury are increasing or decreasing.[10] This is obviously an extremely important deficiency of data systems for developing policy, for planning and for prevention.

Exposure to risk

The other important building block for rates is a measure of population exposure to the hazards that resulted in the injuries counted in the numerator of the rate. For example, if we are interested in the rate of occurrence of road traffic accident (RTA) related injuries, then it might be reasonable to use the number in the target population as a crude measure of exposure. This is because almost everyone is exposed to hazards on the road at some time. However, if this is disaggregated by cause, it will be seen that, amongst children, injury mortality rates for pedestrians and cyclists have reduced. This is due, at least in part, to a reduction in the time a child spends as a pedestrian or a cyclist. From surveys, we know that exposure of these vulnerable road users has changed markedly in the last 30 years. To make sense of these data, we need to be able to relate occurrence of injury to an accurate indicator of exposure to traffic, in this case the time the child spends either walking or cycling on roads.[11]

An important extension of such data is to document the population exposure to known avoidable injury hazards (for example, car passengers without seatbelts). This implies that successful injury surveillance systems must include the evidence base of proven effective forms of injury prevention.

Disablement resulting from improved survival

Existing data suggest that mortality rates are reducing over time for most age groups. We have already seen that some of this will be due to reduced exposure to risk. Additionally, some will be due to the implementation of effective methods of prevention.

A third reason is that the likelihood of survival following an event that results in severe injury has improved.[12] This being the case, then it is likely to follow that there has been an increase in the number of people with disablement. We can only speculate that this is the case, however, since currently we do not have any routinely collected data in the UK that provides an accurate picture of either the magnitude or the nature of the disablement resulting from injury. This is a major deficiency.

The building blocks — current UK national injury data systems

Listed in table 7 are the various injury data systems currently in use in the UK.

Underlying weaknesses in present UK injury data

These major data systems are uncoordinated. It is quite possible for one seriously injured person to generate four sets of unlinked records in different systems. Conversely, relevant injury events or circumstantial data may be required by one system, yet known only to others. Last year the Chief Medical Officer called for the NHS to develop a unified mechanism for the analysis of failures, mistakes, errors and near-misses across the health service, with the aim of providing a single focal point for NHS information on adverse events that was spread across nearly 1,000 different organisations.[14] This has resulted in plans for the establishment of a new agency, the National Patient Safety Agency.[15]

The systems also achieve incomplete coverage. For instance, STATS19 recordings omit many cyclists and pedestrians with

Table 7: Current UK national* injury data systems

Name of system	Method of data collection	Sponsor	Purpose
Death registration	All coded for underlying cause as well as nature of injury (100%)	Office of National Statistics (ONS)**	Vital statistics
Trauma Audit and Research Network (TARN)	Severe injury case units return standardised data to Manchester Centre (approx. 50% of trauma receiving hospitals)	Department of Health (DoH)	Trauma outcome audit
Hospital Episode Statistics (HES)	Inpatient records coded for diagnosis and cause where injured (100%)	DoH	Hospital administration
STATS19 Data	Police reports of injuries in RTA (100% attempted cover)	Department of the Environment, Transport and the Regions (DETR)	Road safety — monitoring vehicle-related injury
Reporting of Injuries, Diseases and Dangerous Occurrences (RIDDOR)	Employer reports of workplace injuries (1 in 20 samples for further investigation)	Health and Safety Executive (HSE)	Safety at work
Home and Leisure Accident Surveillance System (HASS/LASS)	Interviews with accident and emergency attenders (sample of 18 hospitals)	Department of Trade and Industry (DTI)	Consumer safety — monitoring product-related injury
Health Survey for England (HsurvE)	Interview questionnaire concerning medically attended injuries and injuries causing discomfort for >24 hours (sample)	DoH	Wide ranging health survey

* Home Office fire and crime statistics also include some incomplete data on related injuries. For a more comprehensive account and references to data sources see the PHIS report.[13]

** The Department of Health and the Office of National Statistics cover England and England and Wales respectively. There are equivalent authorities in Wales, Scotland and Northern Ireland.

injuries, even when they are admitted to hospital.[16] Home and Leisure Accident Surveillance System (HASS/LASS) interviewers, working in hospital emergency departments not only deliberately exclude workplace and road injury victims as outside their remit, but also miss any home and leisure injuries managed exclusively by local general practitioners. Trauma Audit and Research Network (TARN) surveillance of very severe injuries does not include the half of trauma deaths that precede hospital care.

Several of the data sources provide very sparse coverage. The Health Survey for England and HASS/LASS are sample surveys intended to provide nationally representative data. There are insufficient interviews conducted to provide even Local or Health Authority comparisons.

Other than the Health Survey for England, none of the systems have minimum severity-based case definitions for injury. The numbers of eligible injuries which are counted may vary for unexpected reasons. For instance, the NHS Direct phone advice service has altered thresholds for emergency attendance at hospital. Secular changes in clinical practice may lead to reductions in hospital length of stay, or even influence the decision to admit certain types of injury (eg head injury protocols).

Only the TARN includes direct measures of relative injury severity amongst cases, yet this is the key both to stable epidemiological case definitions and to estimates of likely future disability. Variations in the patterns of injury severity cannot be detected, even though these might be important outcomes of some forms of injury prevention (eg cycle helmets).

Many of the systems have incomplete or inaccurate coding of important variables. Until recently, there was no indication of external cause in many Hospital Episode Statistics (HES) records for injury hospitalisations. In STATS19 records, incomplete recording of school codes creates difficulties in targeting school safety campaigns.

Two of the systems have inadequate denominators with which to calculate population-based rates of injury. TARN and HASS/LASS are unable to fully identify their catchment populations, despite considerable effort. This difficulty is compounded by a general lack of information across most sources on population exposure to relevant hazards or safety features. Variations in cycling injury rates cannot be properly interpreted without information on the numbers of cyclists. This analysis can be further enhanced by data on the prevalence of helmet wearing amongst the cyclists (as long as this is also known for those who are injured). Equivalent exposure data for consumer products or sports injuries is almost wholly lacking.

The last and most pervasive deficiency in current injury data is the lack of information on long-term injury morbidity. There are no routine sources by which the scale of continuing disability following injury can be documented in the UK. We cannot tell whether improved survival has meant increased disability, nor do we know whether the overall burden of injury in terms of life disabled is increasing or decreasing.

Despite these weaknesses, there are important strengths to build upon. Those managing HASS/LASS and STATS19 data have decades of experience in their use in improving consumer products and road safety. UK Hospital Episode Statistics have rapidly improved with recent quality control initiatives. A recent report from the Royal College of Surgeons of England and the British Orthopaedic Association has encouraged comprehensive national participation in TARN. Virtually all injury deaths are subject to Coroners' Inquest Reports — a major and largely unexploited resource for injury prevention. There is also potential strength in combining the wealth of detail already collected in different systems about some types of injury. What is needed is a strong programme of development and research to build on these foundations and to share this expertise.

Examples of UK local and regional injury surveillance

While the overall pattern of injuries in the population is remarkably consistent, variations between geographical locations can be striking. Even contiguous communities may have marked differences in demographic, social, cultural and environmental characteristics that may interact to result in varying rates, causes and outcomes of injury. Analyses of injury data down to fairly small areas can demonstrate epidemiological differences in injury that have profound preventive implications.

Local injury surveillance systems are ideally placed to generate such highly specific information and, where they exist, community-based groups and professionals rely increasingly on these systems to facilitate the planning and evaluation of local initiatives. Three notable examples in the UK are PHISSCH, CHIRPP and AWISS based in the North of England, Scotland and Wales respectively.

PHISSCH, Newcastle

PHISSCH started in 1994 as a collaborative project between the NHS, police and an academic department of child health. The aim of the system is to generate population-based data on children (0-16 years) in Gateshead who are killed or hospitalised due to an unintentional injury, or who are managed as outpatients with relatively severe injuries.[17] Postal questionnaires are used to ascertain detailed descriptions of the circumstances of injury at differing levels of severity. The focus of interest of PHISSCH is thus the upper part of the injury 'iceberg'.

CHIRPP, Glasgow

CHIRPP has a long track record of success in Canada and in its earlier incarnation in Australia. With the support of Health Canada, CHIRPP was piloted at the Royal Hospital for Sick Children, Yorkhill, Glasgow in 1993 and since then it has become an established routine database. CHIRPP is a stand-alone computerised information system that collects mainly narrative data on all children (0-14 years) presenting to the accident and emergency department.[18]

AWISS, Wales

The University of Wales College of Medicine in association with the Welsh Office[19] established AWISS in 1995. The aim of AWISS is to link data from every accident and emergency department throughout Wales in order to monitor injury rates and evaluate interventions. It is unique in the UK as it is the only injury surveillance system that covers an entire region for all ages and all types of injury.

Each of these systems struggle to maintain their minimal resourcing or fulfil their true potential. In addition, new difficulties for development of these and some national systems are presented by impending confidentiality based restrictions on use of patient data. Urgent legislation may be required to make some forms of (eg severe) injuries 'notifiable' to allow essential public health surveillance.

Other countries' national injury surveillance systems

Several countries around the world, including Canada, Sweden, The Netherlands and Australia, have invested substantial resources to improve their injury data systems. Perhaps the most elaborate effort is evident in the USA. Several initiatives are completed or underway to improve the quality and range of US injury information.

The US equivalent to HASS/LASS, the National Electronic Injury Surveillance System (NEISS), is being extended beyond consumer product injuries to encompass the whole range of injuries managed at the one hundred sample emergency room sites, including motor vehicle and workplace injuries, and all types of intentional injury.

The use of ICD (International Classification of Diseases) external cause coding is mandatory, not only in all US-wide sample hospital activity data systems (IP and OP) and in the national health interview survey, but also in many State based Emergency Room surveillance systems (South Carolina and eight other States). Pilot work is under way to enhance this external cause coding with even more detail, using the International Classification of External Causes of Injury (ICECI), a system also designed to be used with extended NEISS.

For many years, US hospitalisation data has already included enhanced ICD nature of injury coding — ICD9 (clinical modification). These codes allow approximate severity classification of injuries and current work is underway to produce an improved version for ICD10.

The US equivalent of STATS19 — run by the National Highways and Transport Safety Administration — includes severity coding of injuries using the Abbreviated Injury Scale. This is a by-product of a linkage system between the US road safety data and relevant material from ambulance, hospital and coroners' records. This Crash Outcome Data Evaluation System (CODES) is used to compose an account of the resource consequences of transport injuries.

In addition to widespread work in the US National Center for Health Statistics to improve death certification and the use of coroners'/medical examiners' records, there are local multi-disciplinary reviews of most child injury deaths (0-18 years) regardless of cause. Such review teams have operated across all Californian counties since 1980 and in every US State since 1987.

These, and other data systems (the US equivalent to table 7 earlier in this chapter lists 31 federally funded national data systems[20]) are now drawn upon extensively for injury reduction targets in Healthy People 2010,[21] their most recent public health strategy document. This explosion in activity and interest in the use, quality and integration of injury statistics has been greatly facilitated by the creation in 1988 of the Office of Statistics and Programming at the US National Center for Injury Prevention and Control (based at the Centers for Disease Control, Atlanta).

International injury surveillance

No truly global injury surveillance system yet exists although much methodological work that is relevant to injury is currently in progress under the auspices of the World Health Organization Burden of Disease programme, the International Collaborative Effort on Injury Statistics of the US National Institutes of Health, and the European Union (EU). The EU has placed strong emphasis on surveillance in its recently launched Injury Prevention Programme — especially the extended use of consumer product safety data from the European Home and Leisure Accident Surveillance System, to which the UK HASS/LASS system contributes (see Appendix 1).

5

Research & development in injury prevention

Current issues

As part of a review into the use of the NHS research and development levy, the Department of Health funded in 1999 a strategic review of research priorities for 'unintentional' injury.[1] This chapter draws significantly on that work. The strategic review identified the following issues:

- the information infrastructure to describe the size and nature of the problem of injury is poor.

- injury research is grossly under-funded relative to the burden on the NHS and on other services, on individuals and on society when compared with other areas.

- across the spectrum of injury prevention and treatment there are large gaps in our knowledge about which interventions do and do not work. Where research into effective methods of prevention does exist, there are some areas of injury prevention where there is still uncertainty regarding effective methods of implementing these research findings in practice.

- there are extensive research programmes that address particular injury types or settings, for example, road traffic accidents and work or home related injuries, which are the responsibility of government departments. For other injury types or settings, there is no single department responsible and so they tend to 'fall through the gaps'. These are priority areas for future research funding.

• despite the large areas of policy responsibility in Britain, ownership of the injury problem, its solutions, and research is fragmented, so that injury types in some settings are missed, for example, drowning, sports injuries, poisonings and rural injuries.

• international experience has shown that progress in reducing injuries is slowest when the problem falls under the responsibility of a number of different government departments.

• there is a need for a comprehensive approach to injury with more collaborative research at all levels, and across all types of injury, from causation right through to rehabilitation of the injured.[2]

Research process and infrastructure

The Department of Health and the NHS have recognised that the funding of research into unintentional injury has in the past been one of the most neglected areas for preventive action, the commissioning of research and the education and training of health professionals.[3]

Key to redressing the balance of small amounts of research aimed at this huge injury problem is to develop an academic infrastructure that builds capacity to increase the level and quality of research into the cause, prevention, treatment and rehabilitation of injury. There must be capacity to carry through any research agenda and such developments of capacity and capability must be sustainable.

Injury research is a complex, heterogeneous discipline covering epidemiology, research reviews, causation studies, intervention and evaluation. Each of these areas of investigation is part of a research process, the ultimate aim of which is to prevent and control the adverse consequences of unintentional injury (see figure 6).

All unintentional injury research relies on access to good quality data, and the review by Ward and Christie[4] highlighted the deficiency of the current information infrastructure in its ability to describe the size and nature of the injury problem (see chapter 4).

Epidemiological evidence about which population groups are most at risk of which types of unintentional injury is incomplete. Without good epidemiological information it is difficult to develop effective programmes for prevention and control.

Not only are there gaps in our epidemiological knowledge, but there are larger ones in our knowledge about which interventions, both prevention and treatment, do and do not work. These are important areas for further research. There is a need for much detailed specialist knowledge because injuries occur in different settings such as on the road, in the home, whilst playing sport, and at work; they involve different population groups (older people, children, young adults); different types of injury (falls, burns, drowning), all of which require different types of intervention to change behaviour or the environment, or to reduce exposure to the risky situation.

To open up new and larger areas, research gaps need to be identified, programmes devised and sufficient funding committed to projects which extend the boundaries of traditional funding budgets. A clear example of this is the need for new research to develop cost-effectiveness measures including nationally agreed ranges of values for the prevention of death and injury across all injury types, and the development of costing standards and costs over time of prevention, treatment, rehabilitation and care. These, and others, such as the social policy context for injury prevention and control, are large and fundamental areas of research which require leadership and funding. They are unlikely candidates for the relatively modest responsive research programmes which form the majority of research opportunities in Britain.

Figure 6: The research process for unintentional injury

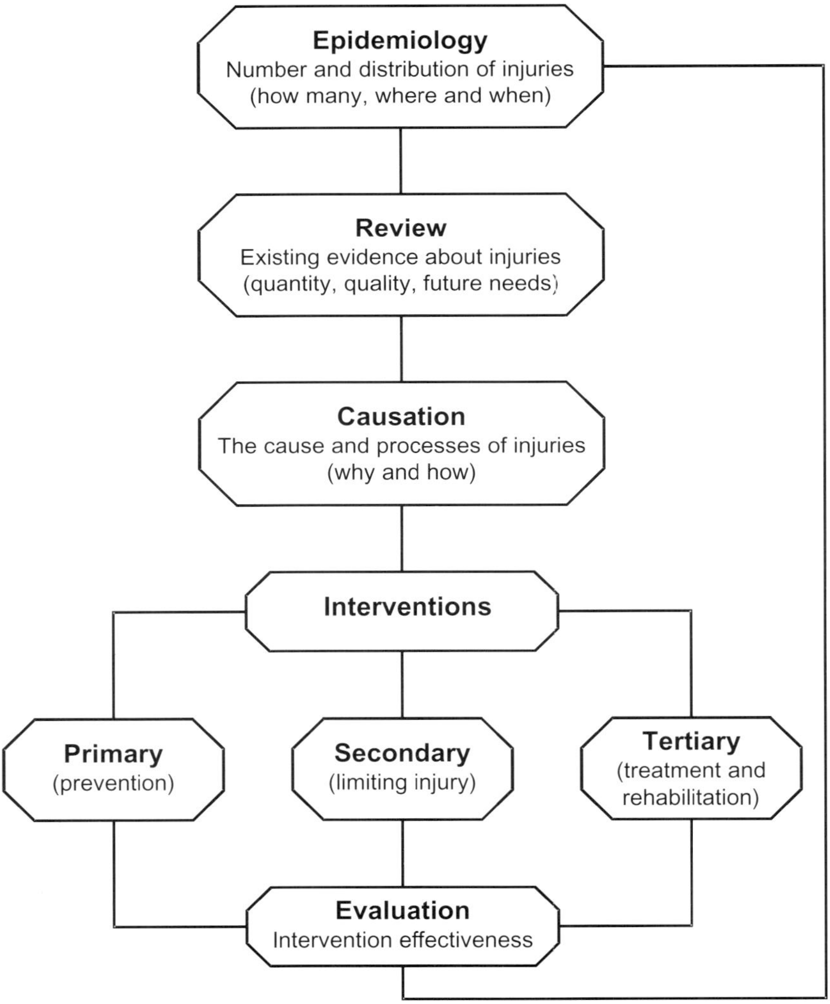

```
                    ┌─────────────────────────────┐
                    │       Epidemiology          │
                    │ Number and distribution of  │──────┐
                    │        injuries             │      │
                    │ (how many, where and when)  │      │
                    └──────────────┬──────────────┘      │
                                   │                      │
                    ┌──────────────┴──────────────┐      │
                    │          Review             │      │
                    │ Existing evidence about     │      │
                    │        injuries             │      │
                    │ (quantity, quality,         │      │
                    │       future needs)         │      │
                    └──────────────┬──────────────┘      │
                                   │                      │
                    ┌──────────────┴──────────────┐      │
                    │         Causation           │      │
                    │ The cause and processes of  │      │
                    │        injuries             │      │
                    │       (why and how)         │      │
                    └──────────────┬──────────────┘      │
                                   │                      │
            ┌────────────┬─────────┴──────────┬───────────┤
            │            │    Interventions   │           │
            │            └────────────────────┘           │
            │                    │                        │
    ┌───────┴────┐      ┌────────┴───────┐      ┌─────────┴──────┐
    │  Primary   │      │   Secondary    │      │    Tertiary    │
    │(prevention)│      │(limiting injury)│      │ (treatment and │
    │            │      │                │      │ rehabilitation)│
    └───────┬────┘      └────────┬───────┘      └─────────┬──────┘
            │                    │                        │
            └──────────┬─────────┴────────────────────────┘
                       │
            ┌──────────┴─────────┐
            │     Evaluation     │
            │ Intervention       │
            │   effectiveness    │
            └────────────────────┘
```

Ownership of the injury problem, its solutions and research is fragmented. There is no lead given by central government and much of the research is through responsive programmes with funding for ideas put forward by individuals or research groups. Ideally there should be a multi-disciplinary academic research programme for each injury type covering everything from epidemiology and basic sciences through to the evaluation of full scale interventions. Where there is collaboration on common issues, expertise should be shared and findings disseminated to all those who have an interest. Academic development is key to addressing this issue. In particular, low levels of funding, combined with ad hoc and short-term research commissioning practice, coupled with poor dissemination, has limited the development of academic infrastructure and capacity.

Research funding

Where central government has taken a commissioning lead on research into unintentional injury, it has resulted in some development of research programmes that address particular injury types or settings. Examples are the research programmes of the Department of the Environment (DETR), the Health and Safety Executive (HSE), the Department of Trade and Industry (DTI) and the Home Office, covering road traffic accidents, work or home related injuries, and fire safety. Funding research programmes in this way can provide a balance covering epidemiology through to evaluation, and helps generate an academic infrastructure and expertise. However, this is patchy (eg there is little epidemiological or economic research on consumer product injuries) and in many areas academic capacity is less well developed.

Unlike cancer research and coronary heart disease, there is virtually no charitable funding for injury research, either through specific dedicated charities, or through more general large scale charitable funding such as The Wellcome Trust.

Of over 50,000 projects registered on the National Research Register (NRR*) (in 1999) approximately 1% was directly related to injury with the majority of this research focused on injury assessment, treatment and rehabilitation, with relatively little being carried out on injury cause and prevention. There was little evidence of collaborative working. This low level of activity is in part a product of the varied commissioning practices of regional offices through which much of the NHS research is commissioned responsively. As a consequence, the academic community carrying out injury prevention research for the Department of Health and the NHS is too small, and difficult to sustain.

Apart from the government departments, other major funders of research include the six research councils, through which much of the academic research is funded. Research into injury prevention, treatment and rehabilitation falls within the remit of the Medical Research Council (MRC). However, only a small number of projects have been funded and the majority deal with the biomedical and clinical consequences of head injury, treatment of severe head and spinal injury, and psychological aspects of rehabilitation. The MRC's programme, Health of the Public,[5] specifically mentioned research topics on unintentional injury in its call for proposals. However, of some 60 projects that were short-listed for further development only two were in the area of injury.

A few projects relevant to injury are also funded by other research councils such as the Engineering and Physical Services Research Council (eg in their Environment and Healthcare

---

* An overview of research on accidental injury funded by the Department of Health, the NHS and the Medical Research Council (MRC) can be obtained from the National Research Register (NRR) and Cochrane databases.

Programme) and the Economic and Social Research Council (Programmes on Risk and Human Behaviour).

In summary, whilst the research councils do fund work into injury, there is no specific stream or programme that targets this area for research. It may be that injury research 'falls through the cracks' but to establish the potential for more targeted funding further discussion with the research councils is essential.

This situation could be changed if central government consolidated its funding streams and commissioning practice and provided a focus for research by forming multi-disciplinary research centres, which in turn could help stimulate sustainable collaborations. Joint funding could address the problems caused by low funding and ad hoc commissioning. Such centres would be instrumental in:

- the development of the academic research workforce capacity to ensure a sufficient supply of senior researchers able to deal with complex methods, work across boundaries and ensure difficult research designs are carried through.

- fostering better understanding among researchers in different disciplines of the variety of valid methodological approaches to answering research questions.

- providing mechanisms for breaking down barriers to effective working by encouraging the building of multi-disciplinary teams who can share and develop research methods as well as share data and research findings.

Additionally, there is a general research role to:

- provide training and guidance to the research community on how to disseminate its research findings so they can be translated into practice. This can be achieved through meetings, virtual networks, dedicated databases of ongoing projects, and journals which recognise unintentional injury as a total concept.

- provide research training to local professionals and encouragement to bid for funds from a variety of funders, both local and national.

- set up a research programme to co-ordinate community and local activities in injury prevention that would facilitate developing strategies for working together and mapping the injury problem across the community.

Research monitoring and information dissemination

At present a focus for this research activity does not exist. It is therefore difficult to identify the expertise and potential opportunities to collaborate with others to provide the right skills mix to address unintentional injury. Expertise on injury tends to be distributed over a wide range of different departments such as psychology, engineering, medicine, and education. Often the expertise is compartmentalised by a specialist skill such as epidemiology, by population group such as older people, or by setting such as road accidents. The situation is not helped by the fact that there is no central register for research on unintentional injury. To avoid duplication of effort the researcher is faced with the daunting task of accessing and interrogating an increasingly wide range of databases including the IRRD (International Road Research Documentation), NRR (National Research Register), COCHRANE, MEDLINE, PSYCHINFO etc.

There is also a problem of knowing what research has taken place, or is in progress, whilst it remains unpublished. Databases of research activity play a key role in informing the research community. The NRR is performing an important role for research funded by the NHS, however, the quality of the information it holds is variable, and it only encompasses a proportion of the research activity in this country. The coverage and quality of information held by research registers needs to be improved.

Although it is hard to locate, it is likely that there is expertise in unintentional injury research that can be shared. Within different regions of the UK there are already clusters of research activity focused on either type of injury or specialist areas.

It is possible that the eight regional NHS Executive offices (London, South East, South and West, Eastern, Trent, West Midlands, Northwest, Northern and Yorkshire) could share this expertise by having inter-region forums on injury research. The Health Development Agency could have a role to play in bringing together this research and helping to disseminate findings as part of its clinical governance role.

Considerable research expertise also exists in the present, and former, public research laboratories such as the Health and Safety Laboratory, the Transport Research Laboratory, the Fire Research Station and the Building Research Establishment. These laboratories have specialist knowledge and skills across the research spectrum through epidemiology to evaluation. More collaborative work between these centres of expertise and other academic organisations is needed.

Dissemination is a key part of putting research into practice. The first step is to make people aware of research findings relevant to their practice. The accessibility of research findings is a major issue across all types of research. Dissemination strategies need to be developed at national, regional and local levels so that research results are accessible and relevant to all those involved in injury prevention no matter what area or type of injury they work in. Research results need to be especially directed to those in health promotion, primary care, social and ambulance services, minor injuries units and other local agencies. One way to achieve this is to ensure that support is given to critical reviews of the science base across the board of injury prevention and treatment, so that what research there is can be made easily accessible to everyone who needs it. A central register of injury research on the Internet would be one way of bringing together and disseminating research from disparate sources.

Dissemination is not just a matter of making people aware of the results of research. It is also about changing professional practice so that those directly or indirectly involved in injury prevention, treatment and care act upon this research evidence. Effective ways need to be developed of getting research into practice across this heterogeneous discipline.

In the USA and Australia, the leading countries in injury prevention initiatives, there is now a large and vibrant injury research community carrying out quality research which is having a major impact on injury prevention, not only in their own countries, but also world-wide. In both cases this was the result of strategic investment decisions in the early 1990s (see Appendix 1).

6

Towards a national policy

Introduction

As previously discussed in this report, injury is one of the most important causes of acute illness, years of life lost and of long-term disability in the UK, and worldwide. It carries one of the highest costs in both human and economic terms and therefore should hold a high government priority. This applies to primary prevention, acute care and rehabilitation. Injury occurs across all life settings (occupational, transport, recreational, educational) and therefore a multiplicity of agencies exist which are accountable in their own area for standards and programmes to monitor and to prevent the occurrence of injury. Internationally, there are different approaches to the co-ordination of injury prevention and control efforts (Appendix 1). A case can be made for co-ordination of injury control efforts both within the health sector and across all sectors of government. The controversial issue of differentiating between a lead agency and a co-ordinating agency has arisen particularly in the USA.

Effective injury prevention relies on multi-agency working at the international, national or local level. No single agency or group of professionals can make all the environmental, engineering, regulatory, enforcement and educational changes needed to bring about reductions in injury. However, there does need to be a focus and responsibility for overall coordination in order to prevent duplication or the overlooking of some areas of injury prevention. This report has highlighted the fragmentation within policy-making structures at all levels, while outlining areas where integration has been achieved. It is evident that greater strategic integration of policy-making structures and responsibilities would be greatly beneficial in terms of cost-effectiveness and impact on injury. The effectiveness of injury policy is therefore heavily dependent on an approach that integrates strategic planning, co-ordination, and implementation across the spectrum and between the international, national and local levels.

UK policy structures for injury prevention

Before the 1997 general election, responsibility for injury prevention lay within eleven government departments and the lack of intra-government co-operation was a significant obstacle to effective decision-making. Since then, there have been efforts to promote cross-departmental working, but also a greater devolution of responsibilities to the Scottish Parliament and Welsh and Northern Ireland Assemblies.

Devolution has changed the way in which the UK is governed. Consumer safety and occupational health and safety are 'retained powers' and remain a UK-wide responsibility, as do some forms of transport, particularly the motorway and rail system, and most taxation and public spending decisions. Devolved responsibilities include health, education, most environmental and local government issues, crime prevention and community safety.

Health policies

Health is a devolved power. The Department of Health has become an English department with an English Public Health Minister. In Scotland, the Scottish Executive has a Health and

Community Minister; in Wales, there is a Minister for Health and Social Services and in Northern Ireland a Minister for Health, Social Services and Public Safety.

In all four health administrations, there is a separation between the health aspects of intentional and unintentional injury. The first is seen nationally as a social care issue and locally as a local government responsibility; the latter is seen as a public health and health service responsibility. In both cases, other departments also take a lead but health professionals are viewed as having a role in the reporting and treatment of injury. The two sides of the health administration, in the main, work independently and separately with other government departments.

Measured in terms of priorities and dedicated resources, intentional injury is a greater priority than unintentional injury. For example, within the Department of Health in England, intentional injury to children and other vulnerable groups is a major issue for the Social Care Group and was a major plank in the White Paper, Modernising social services.[1] Particularly in the child protection field there has been a concerted attempt to ensure co-ordination between different agencies. For example, in April 2000, the Scottish Executive set up a Joint Futures Group to examine how social services and health can work in a more united way. In England, the Department of Health issued guidance in 1999[2] which provides a national framework within which agencies at local level must agree ways of working together. Area Child Protection Committees (ACPCs) have to be set up to cover every local authority area. Where health authority and police boundaries are not coterminous, ACPCs should cover more than one local authority or neighbouring committees should adopt common procedures and protocols.

Protecting children and vulnerable groups from unintentional injury was a major feature in the White Paper, Saving lives: Our healthier nation[3] and included in Towards a healthier Scotland,[4] and Better health, better Wales.[5] However, tackling unintentional injuries was not mentioned in the NHS Plan. In England, a national target has been set to reduce the death rates from accidents by at least one fifth and to reduce the rate of serious injury from accidents by at least one tenth by 2010. An Accident Task Force has been set up. Its remit is to advise the Chief Medical Officer (CMO) on: "the most important priorities for immediate action in order to meet the targets in the White Paper, the development of an implementation plan, whether the necessary delivery structures are in place to take forward the implementation plan, how progress should be monitored and how to develop and publicise a more unified approach across Government and the NHS".[6] The task force has been asked to report back to the CMO within a year.

However, in terms of staffing within the department, resourcing and the priority given to local action, unintentional injury lags well behind intentional injury. There is no formal structure at any level below the task force. The Health Public Service Agreement, which operates until 2002 has only intentional injury as a specified health outcome. In Northern Ireland, the situation is a little different. A Ministerial Group on Public Health, established a Home Safety Strategy Steering Group in 1999 which drew up an action plan for national and local implementation. It is likely that the Northern Ireland Assembly will take this forward.

Transport and environmental policies

Many aspects of road safety, including national speed limits, driver training and testing and vehicle safety, are reserved to the UK Government. Scottish Ministers and the National Assembly for Wales have concurrent responsibility with the UK government for the promotion of road safety and jointly launched the road safety strategy, Tomorrow's roads: Safer for everyone.[7] Implementation of the strategy will be taken forward by the UK and the devolved administrations. Northern Ireland will have its own road safety strategy.

The BMA has policy aimed at reducing driving impairment through alcohol and other drugs.[8] It recommends that permitted blood alcohol concentration for driving in the UK should be reduced to 50mg/100ml from 80mg/100ml, since accident risk increases with blood alcohol concentration. The BMA report Road transport and health[9] reviewed the health impact of road transport including the burden of road traffic accidents, the influence of vehicle speed and the effects of alcohol use on both drivers and pedestrians. The BMA called for an integrated system, with a reduction in vehicle use, the introduction of new information technology to manage traffic better, more rigorous enforcement of speed limits and reduction of the risk of accidents due to consumption of alcohol, drugs or medicines.

The British road safety strategy has set a new 10-year target to achieve by 2010, compared with the average for 1994-98: a 40% reduction in the number of people killed or seriously injured in road accidents; a 50% reduction in the number of children killed or seriously injured; and a 10% reduction in the slight casualty rate, expressed as the number of people slightly injured per 100 million vehicle kilometres. These targets differ from the 'accident' target in Saving lives: Our healthier nation[10] demonstrating the difficulties of co-ordinating policies across government departments. They also differ from targets proposed by the Royal Commission on Environmental Pollution which suggested in 1994 that Government should encourage cycling by seeking to reduce the risk of death while cycling from four to less that two per 100 million kilometres cycled.[11]

On road safety, the government has explicitly recognised that it cannot achieve the strategy on its own and is promoting partnership at national and local level. Two initiatives in particular may assist this. At national level, a Road Safety Advisory Panel has been established, bringing together the major stakeholders to provide advice to Ministers on road safety policies and to advise on progress towards targets. At a local level, local authorities must conduct a child safety audit to identify needs and priorities.

In terms of the environment, departments have slightly different structures but generally have responsibility for housing and area regeneration, land use planning and building control. All departments, therefore, have powers to influence injury prevention both in relation to intentional injury to women and children perpetrated in the home, and unintentional injury, particularly that caused to children and the elderly through housing design, lack of maintenance and poor planning. To date, this is an under-developed area of public policy. However, in Wales, a Framework for a national housing strategy[12] was launched in April 2000 with recommendations from a special task force on vulnerable households. While the task force concentrated on homelessness, the recommendations also include housing measures to prevent and reduce violence to women and children and open the possibility of further action to reduce unintentional injuries through more responsive housing policies.

Fire, policing and crime prevention policies

The Home Office in England and Wales, the Justice Department in Scotland and the Northern Ireland Office have responsibility for preventing intentional and unintentional injuries through their fire safety, policing and crime prevention strategies.

In relation to fire safety, the Home Office has its own target to reduce the number of unintentional fire-related deaths in the home by 20% over 5 years, and to reduce the number of fires overall. There has been a move towards prevention rather than fire fighting, and community fire safety rather than the fire service acting on its own. The National Community Fire Safety Centre (NCFSC) was established in September 1998 to develop a co-ordinated and sustained national strategy for delivering fire safety awareness and education. The Centre operates within HM Fire Services Inspectorate (HMFSI) and the Home Office Fire and Emergency Planning Directorate (FEPD). In Scotland, there has been a similar move towards community fire safety. In a consultation paper on the fire service, Measuring Up,[13] it has been suggested that the Scottish Executive may place a statutory duty on brigades to run community fire safety programmes.

The Home Office also has responsibility for strategic policing policies, funding of police services, and their performance and measurement. It also collects and publishes data on offences and offenders including road traffic offences. In a new initiative, the police performance indicators cover road safety. Police authorities will be required to report on the number of road traffic collisions involving death or serious injury per 1,000 population in their Best value performance plan each year, and their performance in relation to this data will be assessed by Her Majesty's Inspectorate of Constabulary (HMIC) and Audit Commission as part of their duties.

On violence against women and children, the Home Office has pioneered what may be seen as a model of good practice in relation to multi-agency working. In 1999, the Home Office and the Cabinet Office's Women's Unit produced Living without fear,[14] the government's strategic framework on prevention of violence to women and children. The report emphasised the need for multi-agency working and set out the government's commitment to fund innovative projects to reduce domestic violence. An Inter-departmental Official Group on Violence against Women led the implementation of the strategic framework and multi-agency guidance was produced. The Crime and Disorder Act 1998 placed a requirement on local authorities and police to establish crime and disorder partnerships, which are expected to develop a strategy for addressing violence. More recently, a resource manual for health professionals has been jointly produced with the Department of Health.

Consumer affairs and consumer safety

Consumer affairs and consumer safety are retained powers residing in the Department of Trade and Industry. The Department has a Consumer Affairs Directorate whose aim is to help consumers make well-informed purchases that encourage innovation and competitiveness and to protect them from unsafe products and practice. The Directorate works very closely with the European Union and the Health and Consumer Affairs Directorate-General.

The Directorate organises the collection and dissemination of data as part of the Home and Leisure Accident Surveillance Systems, which are linked to the European Surveillance System. They part-fund the British Standards Institution, particularly the development of consumer representation and the National Association of Citizens Advice Bureaux. The Directorate commissions research and runs public awareness campaigns, for example on falls by the elderly, garden safety and DIY safety.

The Department is also concerned with the enforcement of product standards and fair business standards through its partnerships with the Office of Fair Trading and Trading Standards Officers.

Education and early years

Education, including early years education and care, are devolved powers involving responsibility for safety education within the school curriculum and promotion of the safety of children in early years care. The education structures in Scotland and Northern Ireland differ considerably from those in England and Wales. These differences affect injury prevention initiatives. For example, in Scotland there is a pre-school traffic club run by the Scottish Road Safety Campaign and an established approach to teaching road safety across the curriculum, whereas there is no national traffic club in England and a safety framework is only just being developed as part of the Personal, Social and Health Education Curriculum in England.

In recent years, departments have been co-operating more closely and a number of joint initiatives that include injury prevention have been developed. For example, the 'Sure Start' programme is a joint programme between the departments of Health and Education to provide support for children and families in most need. It is anticipated that 250 local programmes will be running by the end of 2001. One of the measures of performance is a reduction in hospital attendances caused by injury in the home involving children under two years.

Other government departments

In addition to the major departments with a substantial interest in injury prevention, other departments have more limited responsibilities. For example, the Department of Culture, Media and Sports has an interest in play and sports safety and has funded the establishment of a Play Safety Forum as part of its policy. The Treasury has an interest through its control of public spending and the Cabinet Office through its work on social exclusion. The Lord Chancellor's Office also has a specific interest in injury prevention, particularly in relation to domestic violence.

A number of government agencies have responsibilities for injury prevention. The most prominent is the Health and Safety Executive (HSE), headed by the tripartite Health and Safety Commission, which is responsible for promoting occupational safety, farm safety, railway safety, the safety of young workers and the safety of adventure activity centres. In terms of injury related research, the HSE probably spends more than all of the government departments mentioned above, despite its narrow remit. The HSE has also published separate targets for reduction in work related injury incidence and lost work days.[15]

The health promotion organisations in England, Scotland and Wales undertake a wide range of public health programmes and initiatives. They have a general responsibility for promoting accident prevention. Recently the agencies have lowered the priority they accord to injury prevention.

The Office for National Statistics and the newly constituted Statistics Commission have responsibility for providing Ministers, the devolved administrations and the public with data on deaths and other health outcomes including injury.

Non-governmental bodies

In addition to the governmental bodies there are a large number of organisations seeking to influence government policy on injury prevention and which carry out injury prevention initiatives themselves. At international, European and British level the standards-making institutions and their partnership consumer organisations make a major contribution to general and individual product safety. Other organisations include professional groups, such as the British Medical Association (BMA) and the medical Royal Colleges who represent the interests of their members working in areas of injury prevention, but also take a wider interest in injury prevention policies; research and academic bodies such as the Transport Research Laboratory, the Institutes of Child Health, and Schools of Gerontology; advisory groups and committees, such as the Parliamentary All-party Advisory Committee on Transport Safety (PACTS); charities and pressure groups.

The same pattern of fragmentation with few examples of integration is evident among other non-governmental bodies. For example the National Society for the Prevention of Cruelty to

Children (NSPCC), Childline and the Child Accident Prevention Trust (CAPT) focus on children, but on different areas of injury. Help the Aged and Age Concern represent the interests of the elderly on both unintentional and intentional injury, and the Royal Society for the Prevention of Accidents (RoSPA) covers all types of unintentional injury. The major exception is initiatives such as the biennial World Conference on Injury Prevention and Control that covers all areas of injury regardless of intent. The main purpose of the conference is to share research findings and practical experience at international level. However, its potential as a lobbying tool has been recognised. The 1996 conference held in Melbourne adopted what has become known as the 'Melbourne Declaration'. The Declaration called for the World Health Organization, the World Health Assembly, the United Nations, the World Bank and global trade, and consumer safety and transport forums to place injury prevention and control higher on their agendas. It also called for the establishment of world networks and coalitions which bring together the professions, sectors and disciplines for co-operative research and action to reduce injury at the community, national, regional and international levels, and for the supporting technologies which facilitate the rapid transfer of data and information. The Declaration also urged all governments to secure a budget allocation for injury prevention and control.

The need for co-ordination

This report has mapped out where governmental policy-making responsibilities lie at national level. It is by no means a comprehensive picture yet it does show a bewildering array of different responsibilities and initiatives being pursued. The policy-making structures are fragmented with policies on unintentional and intentional injury developed and implemented separately even within the same departments. Within unintentional injuries, policy-making responsibilities are sub-divided by injury location and within intentional injuries, responsibilities are sub-divided by whether the injury is self-harm or violence. This fragmentation limits the scope for learning across initiatives still further, seeking common solutions and creating duplication of work. This must mean that many multi-agency groups and practitioners whose clients are at risk of intentional and unintentional injury have to deal with competing initiatives and guidance.

Progress is being made. For example, the new Road Safety Strategy is a partnership approach, jointly launched by the UK government and devolved administrations, with a Road Safety Advisory Panel set up to advise ministers on the implementation of the strategy. However, the transport departments will also need to develop closer links with the devolved departments in health and education as well as links within their own department to environment and housing, if the strategy is to be implemented in an integrated way. Local multi-agency groups will also need direction, funding and support. Similarly, as mentioned previously, the Department of Health has now convened an Accident Task Force. The Welsh Assembly's Framework for a national housing strategy[12] is another example of how different policy priorities can be co-ordinated and integrated through the use of taskforces and consultation. Again, the real challenge will be the implementation of the Framework.

The Home Office's initiative on the prevention of violence against women provides another useful example of how policy making can be integrated across departments and administrations. It shows the need for an integrated approach to implementation, providing a framework of statutory responsibility, resources, support and guidance.

These examples of intra-governmental and cross-departmental working need to be fostered and more time devoted to disseminating both process and outcome evaluations. However, there remains a need for clearer responsibility for leadership and integration between departments and administrations with respect to injury.

The problem of child injuries specifically, has many features that should enable it to move up the policy agenda provided that its visibility is increased. A number of countries have achieved remarkable successes in reducing child injury mortality and in bringing injuries under some control. The UK, USA, Australia, New Zealand and the Nordic countries stand out because they have begun to identify and address the public health burden posed by injuries. These societies have also demonstrated many features of appropriate policy action, from which other countries can learn: the importance of raising the public profile of injuries; the central role of concerned civil society organisations and the role of research in making the issue visible; and assessing effectiveness of interventions and instituting solutions.[16]

However, without integration and joint learning, policy making in injury prevention will continue to be fragmented, characterised by overlapping responsibilities, with decisions made in one area restricting or even conflicting with decisions taken in another. This cannot be an efficient or cost-effective way for future national policies in injury prevention.

Recommendations

1. We recommend that injury prevention should be recognised as one of the major public health priorities in the UK.

Injury surveillance

2. Injury surveillance centres should be established in each UK home country with a remit to collate, interpret, add value to, and disseminate injury statistics across relevant stakeholders; these surveillance centres should also have a remit for

research and development of new methods of surveillance of injuries and injury risk prevalence.

3. The concept of 'injury' rather than 'accidents' should be recognised by the Department of Health and the NHS. The definition of injury and methods of recording data nationally require a consensus from all stakeholders to include hospital departments, police road traffic accident reports, fire services, the Health and Safety Executive, and others.

4. The health sector should adopt a primary role in the collection of high quality data on injuries and their consequences.

5. A comprehensive injury surveillance system should include data from surveys (especially of vulnerable groups) of exposure to known avoidable hazards (eg dwellings without functioning smoke alarms, child pedestrian exposure to non-traffic calmed roads) and of the population at risk of specific injuries (eg kilometres cycled per person).

6. Injury surveillance should include an account of the population prevalence of injury disability. Future national sample surveys of morbidity and disability should clearly identify those cases attributable to injury (preferably linked to detail of the original injury event).

7. Existing data systems concerning injury maintained by separate agencies should be enhanced and co-ordinated.

   • the accident and emergency minimum data set should be made mandatory and be consolidated into an accessible national database. Data collection in primary health care should also provide an important subset of the overall picture since minor injuries frequently present in general practice settings as well as accident and emergency units.

- the national sample system of accident and emergency attenders with home and leisure injuries run by the Department of Trade and Industry (HASS/LASS) should be extended to cover all injury types regardless of circumstances or intent.

- national data concerning road traffic accidents (STATS 19) collated by the Department of the Environment, Transport and the Regions should be developed to include a standardised definition of injury severity and be linked to accident and emergency departments.

- data from coroners' inquest reports relating to injury should be compiled into an anonymous standardised national database.

- each of these injury surveillance systems should include coding of injury circumstances using ICD cause codes and a measure of injury severity using the injury severity score.

8. Consideration should be given by the government to placing a levy on insurance companies to fund research into accident prevention and interventions, and for insurance companies to provide mandatory anonymised reports about all personal injury claims in order to assist in injury surveillance. Investigations should be conducted to ascertain how this can be successfully achieved and implemented as policy.

Research and development

9. The total research spending on injury should be increased to a level commensurate with other major public health problems and positive discrimination should be exercised to balance the lack of charitable and private resourcing. A comprehensive, public, and fully costed account should be kept of all research on injury (public and private/voluntary funded).

10. Systematic efforts are needed to improve the evidence base for effective injury prevention, especially for neglected areas such as intentional injury, sports injury and falls, and to ensure that any widely implemented injury prevention actions for which there is no current evidence of effect are subject to urgent formal trials.

11. New research strategies are needed to:

    • extend the evidence base for effective injury prevention to include details of cost-effectiveness.

    • understand and reverse social inequality in injury risk.

    • develop a national plan for multi-disciplinary injury prevention research including research councils, government departments and other major research funders.

12. There should be several multi-disciplinary injury research centres based in UK universities, covering between them the full range of injury by age group, intent and injury phase from prevention through to rehabilitation.

13. The work of, and data emanating from, the present and former public research laboratories (health and safety, transport research, fire research, building research) should be linked to multi-disciplinary injury research centres.

Implementation and strategic policy development

14. Co-ordinated multi-sectoral action should be focused on the full implementation of those few injury prevention methods for which there is strong evidence of effect (eg car occupant restraints, traffic calming, road speed limit enforcement, smoke alarms, and child proof closures).

15. Further effort is needed to identify and eradicate avoidable mortality and morbidity due to inadequacies in trauma management.

16. A programme budget should be developed to describe the extent of public investment in safety and injury prevention for comparison with other major public health programmes and for audit against cost-effective best practice.

17. The NHS should increase its commitment to health impact assessment and to enforcing health and safety legislation, especially by:

    • encouraging systems for managing health at work.

    • developing occupational health services and competencies.

    • improving data on occupational disease and injury.

    • promoting health and safety in the workplace.

18. An accurate account should be created of the burden of injury versus other major public health threats in the UK using internationally recognised methods such as Disability Adjusted Life Years (DALYs).

19. The four UK health administrations should jointly review and compare the resources and priorities that they give to injury prevention, and identify any specific approaches that have been shown to be effective.

20. A national agency should be established in each of the four home countries following a process of consultation and review with all interested stakeholders with the following remit:

    • establish a single over-arching national body for injury prevention and control working in partnership across government departments.

    • co-ordinate initiatives across all forms of injury, age groups, and at all levels.

- be responsible for establishing national injury surveillance systems.

- commission several multi-disciplinary academic research centres.

- develop a national strategic plan for injury prevention.

- be answerable to a single responsible government minister.

Appendix 1: International approaches to injury control

Introduction

This appendix summarises the World Health Organization and European Union policies for injury prevention and reviews three contrasting national models from the USA, Australia and New Zealand. Where evaluation of their performance has occurred it is noted in order to set out the issues to be considered in proposing a plan for national co-ordination of injury control in the UK. There are few published documents in this area. National websites have been searched for the information that forms the basis of the descriptions and, where possible, researchers have been interviewed.

International policy making

At international level, the World Health Organization (WHO) acts as a catalyst for improving health and health systems across the world. The WHO has adopted an integrated approach to safety incorporating violence, self-harm and unintentional injury, in particular promoting the establishment of 'safe communities' — areas where co-ordinated action on injury is pioneered. In 1999, the WHO's Violence and Injury Prevention Unit launched Injury: A leading cause of the global burden of disease,[1] which concluded:

"The time has come to develop effective injury prevention strategies that will decrease the impact of injuries on the health of the world's population".

The International Labour Organization (ILO) has promoted international co-operation on preventing injury through conventions and recommendations on health and safety in employment. Other international bodies, such as UNICEF and the Red Cross have recently begun to take an interest in injury prevention. However, the report of the 27th International Conference of the Red Cross and Red Crescent[2] drew attention to WHO predictions that road accidents would become the third-leading cause of death world-wide by 2020. The International Committee called upon the national Red Cross and Red Crescent Societies to assist governments in formulating and developing policies to improve road safety and reduce the number of accidents. In February 2001, UNICEF devoted its second 'Innocenti Report Card', A league table of child deaths by injury in rich nations, to injury.[3] The report concludes:

"For most of the causes of child injury deaths there are now proven strategies for prevention. In most industrialised countries, those strategies have yet to be implemented in a comprehensive and consistent way and with a well-informed emphasis on those most at risk".

European Union

The European Union influences national injury prevention policies and regulations in a number of ways. Directives, particularly in the occupational health and safety field, directly affect the rights and responsibilities of organisations, employers and workers at national level. Funding for programmes, such as the European Home and Leisure Accident Surveillance System, affect national programmes and are intended to encourage co-operation and sharing of best practice across Europe. Controls on the import and sale of products, the European system of standard setting and their enforcement have had a major impact on the safety of products sold in national countries.

Within the European Commission, there are three main Directorate-Generals whose work includes injury prevention matters: Employment and Social Affairs, Energy and Transport, and Health and Consumer Affairs Directorates. The Employment and Social Affairs Directorate-General is charged with the development and implementation of standards and regulation on health and safety of work. EU Directives cover the health and safety of those in employment and young workers on placement or in part-time work. The Energy and Transport Directorate-General, whose brief includes energy and the European transport network, funds European-wide road safety programmes. The programme launched in 1993 included the establishment of a European database on road accidents. In the 1997-2001 action programme, the Commission sought to adopt what it describes as an 'ambitious', more integrated approach to safety, with a three-pronged programme targeted at information, accident prevention and damage limitation. Among other initiatives supported as part of this programme, the Commission together with five governments, motoring and consumer organisations have supported the European New Car Assessment Programme (EURO-NCAP) to provide consumers with information on the safety performance of new cars.

The United States of America

Co-ordination of injury control at a national level in the United States of America

Injury control co-ordination exists at several levels within the United States of America including the national, the State and frequently at the county or municipality level.[4]

As a result of the publication of the report by the National Academy of Science in 1985,[5] the Centers for Disease Control (CDC) were given the remit to expand their ongoing activities in injury surveillance and injury prevention. In 1987 they sponsored a national conference. The Injury Control Act of 1990 authorised the CDC to "work in co-operation with other Federal agencies, and with public and non-profit private entities, to promote injury control". It later established the National Centre for Injury Prevention and Control (NCIPC) in 1992.[6] The NCIPC provides "a focal point for the establishment and implementation of national policy related to the prevention and control of non-occupational injuries and violence"[7] (The National Institute of Occupational Safety and Health provides the lead for occupational injury). The NCIPC works closely with other federal agencies who have a remit with regard to injury occurrence. It also holds the lead responsibility for surveillance of injuries.

State injury prevention co-ordination

Most States have established injury control or injury prevention sections within the State Department of Health. The CDC has established relationships to State injury epidemiology or control efforts, and has documented the extent and variability of the burden of injury within the country and in the State.

Surveillance

The Consumer Product Safety Commission conducts the National Electronic Injury Surveillance System (NEISS) based on reports from 101 hospital accident and emergency departments. The National Highway Traffic Safety Administration conducts the Fatality Analysis Reporting System on all road traffic fatalities and the CDC collates and analyses the State returns on all uniform hospital discharge summaries.

Research

The NCIPC extramural injury research programme funds and monitors research in prevention, acute care, rehabilitation, biomechanics and epidemiology. The NCIPC also maintains an intramural research programme focused primarily on surveillance. They established first five, and later ten, injury research and policy centres at universities around the country spread both geographically and with regard to key areas of injury control (prevention, acute care, or rehabilitation). These centres provide training as well as information. Each injury centre is multi-disciplinary involving public health, epidemiology, law, criminal justice, behavioural and social sciences, biostatistics and biomechanics. The ten centres have stimulated the development of other similar centres at other universities. Research is also funded by the Maternal and Child Health Division of the Public Health Service, by various National Institutes of Health (Ageing, Child Health and Development, Mental Health, Alcohol Abuse and Alcoholism etc) and by the National Highway Traffic Safety Administration and the National Institute of Justice. The NCIPC, is part of the US Public Health Service and is funded by Congress.[8]

Evaluation

Two national evaluations monitoring impact and progress in injury prevention and control have been carried out and published by the National Academy of Science: Injury prevention and control[9] and Reducing the burden of injury.[10] The Burden of injury report in 1999 reviewed the whole decade of work on injury both of the NCIPC and other agencies including the impact on practice as well as on research. The report praised the accomplishments of the decade and argued for expansion of resources and activities as well as greater inter-governmental collaboration. The report put particular emphasis on differentiating between the role of a co-ordinating centre and the role of a lead centre, and noted that all agencies with a remit for an area where injury is an issue must develop and maintain leadership, while the NCIPC could take a lead in co-ordinating and fostering co-operation between these agencies. Other key recommendations noted the positive impact of injury control programmes over the previous decade while calling for increased research in specific areas, for expanded federal technical assistance to States, and for increasing the training programmes for professionals. The report also recommended that the national surveillance systems be expanded (specifically to include intentional mortality and to expand NEISS to include all accident and emergency injuries), and that trauma system research and development be enhanced.

Australia

Co-ordination of injury control at a national level in Australia

In Australia, responsibility for different aspects of injury control is organised in different government portfolios at a Commonwealth level. Similar to the USA, the States and Territories have injury control programmes as well as a national co-ordinating centre.

In 1986 health ministers designated injury prevention and control as a national health priority.[11] They gave the remit to the Commonwealth Department of Health and Aged Care to provide overall leadership in the development of national policy responses to injury. The Injury Prevention Section of the Department focuses on all unintentional injury other than those within the remits of the Australian Transport Safety Bureau and the National Occupational Health and Safety Commission.

National surveillance of injury occurrence

State and Territory governments provide hospital separation information to the Australian Institute of Health and Welfare. This information is supplied to the National Injury Surveillance Unit which undertakes public health surveillance of injury at a national level. This unit engages in all aspects of surveillance, and places special emphasis on analysis and dissemination of information, and on developing injury surveillance methods. The Australian Bureau of Statistics collects and reports on injury mortality information. A set of 20 injury indicators was developed and progress towards this set was reported on at a national level in 1997 by the Australian Institute of Health and Welfare.[12]

Approaches to the national co-ordination of research

In 1997 the National Health and Medical Research Council investigated the status of injury research in Australia. Their report examined the current state of injury research and barriers to future progress. In 1998 an expert committee was established, with the aim of implementing the recommendations of the report, and promoting injury research efforts in Australia. The Injury

Research Committee is currently examining possible priorities and potential partnerships with other stakeholders. These include the Australian Institute of Criminology and academic partners such as the long standing Monash University Accident Research Centre and the new multi-disciplinary Injury Risk Management and Prevention Research Centre at the University of New South Wales (funded by the New South Wales Health Department).[13,14]

State and territorial links

Each Australian State and Territory Department of Health has an Injury Prevention Manager who has a liaison and co-ordination role for certain injury issues within their jurisdiction. As with the Commonwealth, various injury types are the responsibility of other agencies, such as the State Road Safety/Transport Authority, or the State Workcover Authority, the workplace safety system. Queensland and Victoria operate State-based injury surveillance systems.[15,16]

New Zealand

Co-ordination of injury control at a national level in New Zealand

As a result of a commissioned enquiry into injury prevention and compensation in the 1980s, the Accident Compensation Commission was set up initially to provide no fault compensation for injuries, whether they occurred in the home, at work or on the road. This later became the Accident Compensation Corporation, (ACC), which has historically provided the highest level of injury control co-ordination within the country because of its remit to reduce the impact of injury on individuals and the community.

Besides providing insurance, their activities include injury prevention initiatives, co-ordinating case management and rehabilitation services and funding, (together with the New Zealand Medical Research Council, and two internationally renowned injury prevention research centres at the Universities of Auckland and Otago).[17,18] Though there had been a diminished injury prevention role and a move towards privatisation of insurance in the late 1990s, this was rescinded by legislation in 2000, reaffirming the Corporation's role in prevention and rehabilitation. They have a large central budget for accomplishing their remit which includes prevention, rehabilitation and compensation of two billion NZ dollars, drawn as a levy on the population. There has been no formal evaluation of the work of the ACC; although costs have come down and claims have decreased throughout its tenure. This is thought informally to be a result of decreased injury occurrence, changing criteria for compensation and the provision of more effective rehabilitation.[19] As in the USA and Australia the enforcement of Transport and Occupational Safety legislation lie with the remit of separate agencies.

Summary

- The three models highlighted, (USA, Australia and New Zealand) illustrate different approaches to the provision of injury control at varying stages of development.

- Though all three countries have separate government agencies with a remit for injury prevention within their sector, historically there has been substantial development of an inter-governmental co-ordinating function especially in the USA and in Australia.

- In regard to national surveillance, the NCIPC in the USA and the Australian NISU have a co-ordinating role, but separate agencies still maintain surveillance systems related to their individual remits. These control units also undertake primary research on injury surveillance methods.

- The NCIPC in the USA and the ACC in New Zealand both have a role in funding multi-disciplinary injury control research centres. In Australia the Monash University Accident Research Centre and the new centre at the University of New South Wales are supported by the State Health Departments. Competitive funding for other research grants within National Institutes of Health or Research Councils does not appear to generate much injury prevention research.

- In terms of funding, New Zealand has the most innovative system linking the funding for prevention to the budget for injury compensation. A similar system is operated by the Traffic Accident Commission in Victoria State, Australia. A recent evaluation of the programme in the USA argues for expanding the activities of the national agencies involved in injury control.

References

Chapter 1

1   British Medical Association. *A BMA guide to living with risk*. London: Penguin Books, 1990

2   Pless I, Towner E, eds. Action on Injury. Setting the agenda for children and young people in the UK. *Injury Prevention: Special Supplement* 1998;4(4)

3   Department of Health. *Our healthier nation*. London: The Stationery Office, 1998

4   British Medical Association. *Growing up in Britain: Ensuring a health future for our children*. London: BMJ Books, 1999

5   Royal Society Study Group. *Risk assessment*. London: Royal Society, 1983

6   Health and Safety Commission. *Newsletter 135*. Sudbury: HSC, February 2001

7   British Medical Association. *A code of practice for the safe use and disposal of sharps*. London: BMA, 1990

8   British Medical Association. *Stress and the medical profession*. London: BMA, 1992

9   British Medical Association. *Environmental and occupational risks of health care*. London: BMA, 1994

10 British Medical Association. *Morbidity and mortality of doctors*. London: BMA, 1993

11 European Centre on Health of Societies in Transition, London School of Hygiene and Tropical Medicine. *Childhood injuries in industrialised countries*. A project commissioned by UNICEF Innocenti Research Centre. June 2000

Chapter 2

1   Krug E. Injury: *A leading cause of the global burden of disease*. Geneva: World Health Organization, 1999

2   Murray CL, Lopez AD. Alternative projections of mortality and disability by cause 1990-2020: Global burden of disease study. *The Lancet*, 1997;349:1498-504

3   Purdon S. *Non-fatal accidents. Health Survey for England 1996.* London: The Stationery Office, 1998

4   NHS Executive. *Burdens of disease - a discussion document.* London: Department of Health, 1996

5   Department of Health. *Saving lives: Our healthier nation.* London: The Stationery Office, 1999

6   Department of Health and Social Security. *Health and well-being into the next millennium. Regional strategy for health and social wellbeing 1997-2002.* Belfast: Department of Health and Social Services. (http://www.dhssni.gov.uk/publications/archived/health.htm)

7   The Scottish Office Department of Health. *Towards a healthier Scotland.* Edinburgh: The Stationery Office, 1999

8   The Welsh Office. *Better health - Better Wales: Strategic framework.* London: The Stationery Office, 1998

9   Department of Health and Social Security. *Health and well-being into the next millennium. Regional strategy for health and social wellbeing 1997-2002.* Belfast: Department of Health and Social Services. (http://www.dhssni.gov.uk/publications/archived/health.htm)

10   The Scottish Office Department of Health. *Towards a healthier Scotland.* Edinburgh: The Stationery Office, 1999

11   Krug E. *Injury: A leading cause of the global burden of disease.* Geneva: World Health Organization, 1999

12   Petridou E. Childhood injuries in the European Union: Can epidemiology contribute to their control? *Acta Paediatrica,* in press

13   Information Division, Department of Health, London. *Personal Communication,* 2000

14   Information Statistics Division, Edinburgh. *Personal Communication,* 2000

15   General Registrar Office, Belfast, mid-year population estimates 1991 and 1996 + abstract of cause of death at different age periods. *Personal Communication,* 2000

16   DiGuiseppi C, Roberts I, Li L. Influence of changing travel patterns on child death rates from injury: Trend analysis. *BMJ* 1997;314:710

17   Roberts I, DiGuiseppi C, Ward H. Childhood injuries: Extent of the problem, epidemiological trends, and costs. *Injury Prevention: Special Supplement* 1998;4:S10-6

18   Office for National Statistics. *Health inequalities: Decennial supplement.* London: The Stationery Office, 1997

19   Office for National Statistics. Mortality data. *Personal Communication,* 2000

20   Office for National Statistics. Hospital Episode Statistics 1998. Personal
      Communication, 2000

21   McCormick A, Fleming D, Charlton J. *Morbidity statistics from general practice. Fourth
      national study 1991-2.* Series MB5 No 3 OPCS. London: HMSO, 1995

22   Purdon S. *Non-fatal accidents. Health Survey for England 1996.* London: The Stationery
      Office, 1998

23   Department of Trade and Industry. *Home accident surveillance system including leisure
      activities.* London: Department of Trade and Industry, 2000

24   McCormick A, Fleming D, Charlton J. *Morbidity statistics from general practice. Fourth
      national study 1991-2.* Series MB5 No 3 OPCS. London: HMSO, 1995

25   Airey CM, Chell S, Tennant A *et al.* Epidemiology of disability and occupational
      handicap amongst survivors of major trauma. *Disability and Rehabilitation,* "scheduled
      for" 2001;23:509-15

26   Rigby A, Airey M, Tennent A *et al* The effect of post-traumatic stress symptoms and
      disability status on quality of life: findings in a major trauma survivor cohort at five years.
      Personal Communication, 2000

27   Mirrlees-Black C, Mayhew P, Percy A. *The 1996 British Crime Survey Home Office
      Statistical Bulletin* 1996;19:27-36

28   Office of National Statistics. Road accidents, vehicles involved and casualties. *Annual
      Abstract of Statistics.* London: The Stationery Office, 2000

29   Department of the Environment, Transport and the Regions. *Highways Economic Note
      No. 1,* 1999

30   Department of Trade and Industry. *Home accident surveillance system including leisure
      activities.* London: Department of Trade and Industry, 2000

31   Office of National Statistics. Road accidents, vehicles involved and casualties. *Annual
      Abstract of Statistics.* London: The Stationery Office, 2000

32   Sharples PM, Storey A, Aynsley-Green A *et al.* Causes of fatal childhood accidents
      involving head injury in northern region 1979-86. *BMJ* 1990;301:1193-7

33   Cryer C. Reducing accidental injuries among older people in England. *Personal
      Communication, 2000*

34   Bandolier. *Injuries from falls are increasing in older adults.* Bandolier 15 May 2001
      (http://www.jr2.ox.ac.uk/Bandolier/band66/b66-3.html)

35   Trunkey DD, Lim RC. Analysis of 425 consecutive trauma fatalities: An autopsy study.
      Journal of the American College of Emergency Physicians 1974;3:368-71

36   Anderson ID, Woodford M, Irvine MH. Preventability of death from penetrating injury in
      England and Wales. *Injury* 1989;20:69-71

37 Roberts I, Campbell F, Hollis S *et al.* Reducing accident death rates in children and young adults: The contribution of hospital care. Steering Committee of the Major Trauma Outcome Study Group. *BMJ* 1996:313:1239-41

38 Lecky F, Woodford M. Yates DW. Trends in trauma care in England and Wales 1987-97. UK Trauma Audit and Research Network. *The Lancet* 2000;355:1771-5

39 The Royal College of Surgeons of England. *Better care for the severely injured. A joint report from the Royal College of Surgeons of England and the British Orthopaedic Association.* The Royal College of Surgeons of England: Hampshire, 2000

40 King's Fund and Audit Commission. *Trends in rehabilitation policy: A review of the literature.* London: King's Fund, 1998

41 Royal College of Physicians. *Medical rehabilitation for people with physical and complex disabilities. A report from the Royal College of Physicians Committee on rehabilitation medicine.* London: Royal College of Physicians, 2000

42 Gentleman D. Improving outcome after traumatic brain injury - progress and challenges. *British Medical Bulletin* 1999;55:910-26

43 Barnes MP. Rehabilitation after traumatic brain injury. *British Medical Bulletin* 1999;55:927-43

44 Haddon W. Advances in the epidemiology of injuries as a basis for public policy. *Public Health Reports* 1980;95:411-2

45 Maycock G. *Drinking and driving in Great Britain - a review.* Transport Research Laboratory Report 232. Crowthorne: Transport Research Laboratory, 1997

46 Murray CL, Lopez AD. Alternative projections of mortality and disability by cause 1990-2020: Global burden of disease study. *The Lancet* 1997;349:1498-504

47 Department of Health and Social Security. *Health and well-being into the next millennium. Regional strategy for health and social wellbeing 1997-2002.* Belfast: Department of Health and Social Services. (http://www.dhssni.gov.uk/publications/archived/health.htm)

48 The Scottish Office Department of Health. *Towards a healthier Scotland.* Edinburgh: The Stationery Office, 1999

49 Sibert JR, Craft AW, Jackson RH. Child-resistant packaging and accidental child poisoning *The Lancet* 1977;2(8032):289-90

50 Towner E, Dowswell T, Mackereth C *et al. What works in preventing unintentional injuries in children and adolescents? An updated systematic review.* London: Health Development Agency, 2001

51 Erdmann TC, Feldman KW, Rivara FP *et al.* Tap water burn prevention: The effect of legislation. *Paediatrics* 1991;88:572-7

52 Speigel CN, Lindaman FC. Children can't fly: a program to prevent childhood morbidity and mortality from window falls. *American Journal of Public Health* 1977;67:1143-7

53 Runyan CW, Bangdiwala SI, Linser MA *et al*. Risk factors for fatal residential fires. *New England Journal of Medicine* 1992;327:859-63

54 Mallonee S, Istre GR, Rosenberg M *et al*. Surveillance and prevention of residential-fire injuries. *New England Journal of Medicine* 1996;335:27-31

55 Roberts I. Smoke alarm use: Prevalence and household predictors. *Injury Prevention* 1996;2:263-5

56 DiGuiseppi C, Slater S, Roberts I *et al*. The 'Let's Get Alarmed!' initiative: A smoke alarm give-away programme. *Injury Prevention* 1999;5:177-82

57 Bly P, Dix M, Stephenson C. *Comparative study of European child pedestrian exposure and accidents. A research report to the Department of the Environment, Transport and the Regions.* Norwich: The Stationery Office, 1999

58 Towner E, Dowswell T, Simpson G *et al*. *Health promotion in childhood and young adolescence for the prevention of unintentional injuries. Health promotion effectiveness reviews.* London: Health Education Authority, 1996

59 Mackie AM, Ward HH, Walker RT. *Urban Safety Project 3. Overall evaluation of area wide schemes.* Transport and Road Research Laboratory Report 263. Crowthorne: Transport and Road Research Laboratory, 1990

60 Webster DC, Mackie AM. *Review of traffic calming schemes in 20 mph zones.* Transport Research Laboratory Report 215. Crowthorne: Transport Research Laboratory, 1996

61 Kimber R. Appropriate speeds for different road conditions. In: Parliamentary Advisory Council for Transport Safety. *Speed, accidents and injury: Reducing the risks.* London: PACTS, 1990

62 Coleman P, Munro J, Nicholl J *et al*. *The effectiveness of interventions to prevent accidental injury to young persons aged 15-24 years: A review of the evidence.* University of Sheffield: Medical Care Research Unit, 1996

63 Somers RL. On the cost of repealing motorcycle helmet laws. *American Journal of Public Health* 1983;73:1216

64 Chenier TC, Evans L. Motorcyclist fatalities and the repeal of mandatory helmet wearing laws. *Accident Analysis and Prevention* 1987;19:133-9

65 Thompson DC, Rivara FP, Thompson R. Helmets for preventing facial injuries in bicyclists. *Cochrane Database of Systematic reviews*, Issue 2, 2000

66 Coleman P, Munro J, Nicholl J *et al*. *The effectiveness of interventions to prevent accidental injury to young persons aged 15-24 years: A review of the evidence.* University of Sheffield: Medical Care Research Unit, 1996

67   Pepersack T. Falls in elderly persons: Evaluation of risk and prevention. *Revue Medicale de Bruxelles* 1997;18:227-30

68   Campbell AJ, Robertson MC, Gardner MM *et al*. Psychotropic medication withdrawal and a home-based exercise program to prevent falls: A randomised controlled trial. *Journal of the American Geriatrics Society* 1999;47:850-3

69   Gillespie LD, Gillespie WJ, Cumming R *et al*. Interventions for preventing falls in the elderly. *Cochrane Database of Systematic Reviews,* Issue 1, 2000

70   Close J, Ellis M, Hooper R *et al*. Prevention of falls in the elderly trial (PROFET): A randomised controlled trial. *The Lancet* 1999;353:93-7

71   Feder G, Cryer C, Donovan S *et al*. *Guidelines for the prevention of falls in older people.* London: Dept of General Practice and Primary Care, Queen Mary and Westfield College, 2000

72   Gunnell D, Frankel S. Prevention of suicide: Aspiration and evidence. *BMJ* 1994;308:1227-33

73   Nicholl J. Optimal use of resources for treatment and prevention of injuries. *British Medical Bulletin* 1999;55:713-25

74   Department of Health. *National service framework for mental health services in England: Modern standards and service models for mental health.* London: Department of Health, 1999

75   Roberts I, Kramer MS, Suissa S. Does home visiting prevent childhood injury? A systematic review of randomised controlled trials. *BMJ* 1996;312:29-33

76   British Medical Association. Childhood injury and abuse In: *Growing up in Britain: Ensuring a healthy future for our children.* London: BMA, 1999

77   Dinh-Zarr T, DiGuiseppi C, Heitman E *et al*. Interventions for preventing injuries in problem drinkers. *Cochrane Database of Systematic Reviews,* Issue 1, 2000

78   Gergen KJ & Gergen MM. *Social Psychology.* New York: Harcourt Brace Jovanovich, 1981

79   Metropolitan Police Football Intelligence Unit www.met.police.uk/publicorder/football_intelligence.htm

80   Health and Safety Executive. *Managing crowds safety* HS(G)154. London: HMSO, 1996

81   Jackson R, Towner E. Report on socio-economic influences on unintentional injury in childhood. A discussion document prepared for the Child Accident Prevention Trust. London: CAPT 1997. *Personal Communication*, 2000

82   Colver A, Hutchinson P, Judson C. Promoting children's home safety. *BMJ* 1982;285:1177-80

83   DiGuiseppi C, Slater S, Roberts I *et al*. The 'Let's Get Alarmed!' initiative: A smoke alarm give-away programme. *Injury Prevention* 1999;5:177-82

84 Acheson D. *Independent inquiry into inequalities in health* (The Acheson Report). London: The Stationery Office, 1998

85 Marland R. Keep your seat - save your life. *Archives of environmental health* 1967;15:1-2

86 Scott PP, Willis PA. *Road casualties in Great Britain during the first year with seat-belt legislation.* Transport Research Laboratory Report 9. Crowthorne: Transport and Road Research Laboratory, 1985

87 Department of Health. *Saving lives: Our healthier nation.* London: The Stationery Office, 1999

88 Department of Health. *National service framework for older people: Modern standards and service models for mental health.* London: Department of Health, 2001

89 Department of Health. *National service framework for mental health services in England: Modern standards and service models for mental health.* London: Department of Health, 1999

90 Executive Letter. *Health Action Zones - an invitation to bid* EL (97) 65. London: Department of Health, 1997

91 Health Service Circular. *Healthy living centres* HSC1999/008. London: Department of Health, 1999

Chapter 3

1 Ward H, Christie N. *Strategic review of research priorities for accidental injury.* London: University College of London/Transport Research Laboratory, 2000

2 Gross C, Anderson G, Powe N. The relation between funding by the National Institute of Health and the burden of disease. *New England Journal of Medicine* 1999;340:1881-7

3 Baker S, O'Neill B, Ginsburgh M *et al. Trends in mortality from injuries and other causes. The injury fact book (3rd ed.Vol 10-16).* Oxford: Oxford University Press, 1992

4 Barss P, Smith G, Baker S, *et al. Injury prevention - an international perspective (epidemiology, surveillance and policy).* Oxford: Oxford University Press, 1998

5 Miller P. Costs of injury by major cause, US 1995. In: Mulder S, van Beeck E, eds. *Measuring the burden of injuries.* Noordwijkerhout: European Consumer Safety Association (ECOSA), 1998

6 Miller T, Romano E, Spicer R. The cost of childhood unintentional injuries and the value of prevention. *Unintentional injuries in childhood: The future of children* 2000;10:137-62

7 Danseco E, Miller T, Spicer R. Incidence and costs of 1987-1994 childhood injuries: Demographic breakdowns. *Pediatrics* 2000;105:E271-8

8   Hygeia Group, Angus D, Cloutiere A, *et al. Smart risk - the economic burden of unintentional injury in Canada: A summary.* Ontario:Gov.Ontario, 1998

9   Watson W, Ozanne-Smith J. *The cost of injury to Victoria.* Victoria, Australia: Monash University Accident Research Centre, 1997

10   Phillips DE, Langley JD, Marshall SW. Injury: The medical and related costs in New Zealand 1990. *New Zealand Medical Journal* 1993;106:215-8

11   Kramer P. A first estimate for The Netherlands based on the DALY approach. In: Mulder S, Van Beeck E, eds. *Measuring the burden of injury.* Noordwijkerhout: European Consumer Association (ECOSA), 1998

12   NHS Executive. *Burdens of disease - a discussion document.* London: Department of Health, 1996

13   Ward H, Christie N. *Strategic review of research priorities for accidental injury.* London: University College of London/Transport Research Laboratory, 2000

14   Roberts I, DiGuiseppi C, Ward H. Childhood injuries: Extent of the problem, epidemiological trends and costs. *Injury Prevention: Special Supplement* 1998;4:S10-S16

15   Miller P. Costs of injury by major cause, US 1995. In: Mulder S, van Beeck E, eds. *Measuring the burden of injuries.* Noordwijkerhout: European Consumer Safety Association (ECOSA), 1998

16   NHS Executive. *Burdens of disease - a discussion document.* London: Department of Health, 1996

17   Ward H, Christie N. *Strategic review of research priorities for accidental injury.* London: University College of London/Transport Research Laboratory, 2000

18   Roberts I, DiGuiseppi C, Ward H. Childhood injuries: Extent of the problem, epidemiological trends and costs. *Injury Prevention: Special Supplement* 1998;4:S10-S16

19   European Centre on Health of Societies in Transition, London School of Hygiene and Tropical Medicine. *Childhood injuries in industrialised countries.* A project commissioned by UNICEF Innocenti Research Centre. June 2000

20   Barss P, Smith G, Baker S, *et al. Injury Prevention - an international perspective. (epidemiology, surveillance and policy).* Oxford: Oxford University Press, 1998

21   Murray C, Lopez A. *The global burden of disease.* Geneva: WHO, 1996

22   Krug E. *Injury: A leading cause of the global burden of disease.* Geneva: WHO, 1999

23   Bevan G, Hollinghurst S, Bowie C. Disability Adjusted Life Years: An introduction to their objectives, methods and potential. *EuroHealth* 1999;5:28-30

24   Gross C, Anderson G, Powe N. The relation between funding by the National Institute of Health and the burden of disease. *New England Journal of Medicine* 1999;340:1881-7

25   Baker S, O'Neill B, Ginsburgh M *et al. Trends in mortality from injuries and other causes. The injury fact book (2nd ed. Vol 10-16)*. Oxford: Oxford University Press, 1992.

26   Hygeia Group, Angus D, Cloutiere A, *et al. Smart risk - the economic burden of unintentional injury in Canada: A summary*. Ontario:Gov.Ontario, 1998

27   Watson W, Ozanne-Smith J. *The cost of injury to Victoria*. Victoria, Australia: Monash University Accident Research Centre, 1997

28   Kramer P. A first estimate for The Netherlands based on the DALY approach. In: Mulder S, Van Beeck E, eds. *Measuring the burden of injury*. Noordwijkerhout: European Consumer Association (ECOSA), 1998

29   Committee on Trauma Research, Commission on Life Sciences, National Research Council & Institute of Medicine. *Injury in America: A continuing public health problem*. Washington DC: National Academic Press, 1985

30   Rice D, MacKenzie E. *Cost of injury in the United States. Report to Congress 1989*. San Francisco: Institute for Health and Ageing, University of California; Injury Prevention Center Johns Hopkins University, 1989

31   Bonnie RJ, Fulco CE, Liverman CT. *Reducing the burden of injury: Advancing prevention and treatment*. Washington DC: Institute of Medicine, National Academy Press, 1999

32   Bonnie RJ, Fulco CE, Liverman CT. *Reducing the burden of injury: Advancing prevention and treatment*. Washington DC: Institute of Medicine, National Academy Press, 1999 (Reprinted with permission of the publisher National Academy Press)

33   NCIPC (National Centre for Injury Prevention and Control). *Inventory of federally funded research in injury prevention and control FY 1995*. Atlanta, GA: NCIPC, 1997

34   IOM (Institute of Medicine). *Scientific opportunities and public needs: Improving priority setting and public input at the National Institute of Health*. Washington DC: National Academy Press, 1998

35   NCHS (National Centre for Health Statistics). *Health, United States, 1998 with socioeconomic status and health chartbook*. Hyattsville, MD: NCHS. DHHS Publication No. (PHS) 98-1232, 1998

36   Better Health Commission. *Looking forward to better health*. Canberra: Australian Government Publishing Service: Canberra, 1986

37   World Health Organization Advisory Group. *Investing in health research and development*. Geneva: WHO, 1996: Ad hoc committee on health research relating to future intervention options

38   World Health Organization Advisory Group. *Investing in health research and development*. Geneva: WHO, 1996: Ad hoc committee on health research relating to future intervention options

39   Office for National Statistics. *20th century mortality: 1996-99 update disk*. London: The
      Stationery Office, 1999

40   Murray C, Lopez A. *The global burden of disease*. Geneva: WHO, 1996

41   Murray C, Lopez A. *The global burden of disease*. Geneva: WHO, 1996

42   Hollinghurst S, Bevan G, Bowie C. Estimating the avoidable burden of disease by
      Disability Life Years (DALYs). *Health Care Management Science* 2000;3:9-21

43   Medical Research Council. *Personal communication, 2001*

44   Hartley-Brewer J. Neglect of road safety spending costs lives. *The Guardian* 9 Feb 2000

45   Wiseman V, Mooney G. Burden of illness. Estimates for priority setting. A debate
      revisited. *Health Policy* 1998;43:243-51

46   Williams A. Measuring the burden of disease: What's the use? *EuroHealth* 1999;5:31-3

47   British Medical Association. *Health and Environmental Impact Assessment*. London:
      BMA, 1998

48   Torrance GW. Measurement of health state utilities for economic appraisal. *Journal of
      Health Economics* 1986;6:1-30

49   Mason J, Drummond M, Torrance G. Some guidelines on the use of cost-effectiveness
      league tables. *BMJ* 1993;306:570-2

50   Adapted from Miller T, Romano E, Spicer R. The cost of childhood unintentional injuries
      and the value of prevention. *Future of children.* 2000;10:137-63

51   Boyle M, Torrance G, Sinclair J *et al*. Economic evaluation of neonatal intensive care of
      very low birth weight infants. *New England Journal of Medicine* 1983;308:1330-7

52   Miller T, Levy D. Cost outcome analysis in injury prevention and control: Eighty-four
      recent estimates for the United States. *Medical Care* 2000;38:562-82

53   Tengs T, Adams M, Pliskin JS *et al*. Five hundred life-saving interventions and their
      cost-effectiveness. *Risk Analysis* 1995;15:369-90

54   Department of the Environment, Transport and the Regions. *Highways Economics Note
      No. 1*, 1998

55   Mackie AM, Ward HH, Walker RT. *Urban Safety Project 3. Overall evaluation of area
      wide schemes*. Transport and Road Research Laboratory Report 263. Crowthorne:
      Transport and Road Research Laboratory, 1990

56   Mackenzie J. *The work of the Victoria State Traffic Accident Commission.* Plenary
      presentation. 3rd International Conference on Injury Prevention and Control. Melbourne,
      Australia, 1996

57   World Health Organization. *Global forum for health research 2000 - the 10/90 report on
      health research 2000.* Geneva: WHO, 2000

58   Petridou E. Childhood injuries in the European Union. Can epidemiology contribute to their control? *Acta Paediatrica*, in press

59   Bly P, Dix M, Stephenson C. *Comparative study of European child pedestrian exposure and accidents. A research report to The Department of the Environment, Transport and the Regions.* Norwich: The Stationery Office, 1999

60   Campbell H. High levels of incorrect use of seat belts and child restraints in Fife - an important and under-recognised road safety issue. *Injury Prevention* 1997;3:17-22

61   Towner E, Towner J. Study of effective measures in reducing childhood deaths and serious injuries in 29 OECD countries. *A league table of child deaths by injury in rich nations.* Vol. 13-14. Florence, Italy: UNICEF Innocenti Research Centre, 2001

62   ISCAIP. International smoke detector legislation. *Injury Prevention* 1999;5:254-5

63   DiGuiseppi C, Roberts I, Speirs N. Smoke alarm installation in inner London council housing: cross sectional study. *Archives of Disease in Childhood* 2000;316:904-5

64   Towner E, Ward H. Prevention of injuries to children and young people: The way ahead for the UK. *Injury Prevention: Special supplement* 1998;4:S17-S25

65   Cigarettes (Fire Safety) Bill. *Parliament of New Zealand members' bill introduced by G. Gillon.* November 2000

66   Roberts I, DiGuiseppi C. An international study of the exposure of children to traffic. *Injury Prevention* 1997;3:89-93

67   DiGuiseppi C, Roberts I. Influence on changing travel patterns on child death rate. Injury trend analysis. *BMJ* 1997;314:710-3

68   Hillman M, Adams J, Whitelegg J. *One false move: A study of children's independent mobility.* London: Policy Studies Institute, 1990

69   Safe Kids Survey: reported in *Child Accident Prevention Trust Annual Report 2000.* CAPT: London, 2000

70   British Medical Association. *Cycling: Towards health and safety.* Oxford: Oxford University Press 1992

71   Secretary of State for Health. *Our healthier nation: A contract for health.* Command Paper 3852. Section 2.23. London: The Stationery Office, 1998

72   Goddard G. *Summary fire statistics. United Kingdom 1995 Home Office Statistical Bulletin.* London: Government Statistical Service, 1997

Chapter 4

1   Thacker S, Parrish R, Trowbridge F. A method for evaluating systems of epidemiological surveillance. *World Health Statistics Quarterly* 1988;41:11-18

2   Centers for Disease Control. Guidelines for evaluating surveillance systems. *Mortality and Morbidity Weekly Report* 1988;37:1-18

3   Centers for Disease Control. Guidelines for evaluating surveillance systems. *Mortality and Morbidity Weekly Report* 1988;37:1-18

4   Stone D, Morrison A, Ohn T. Developing injury surveillance in accident and emergency departments. *Archives of Diseases in Childhood* 1998;78:108-110

5   Department of Health. *Saving lives: Our healthier nation.* London: The Stationery Office, 1999

6   Bonnie R, Fulco C, Liverman C. *Reducing the burden of injury - advancing prevention and treatment.* Institute of Medicine Committee on Injury Prevention and Control. Washington DC: National Academy Press, 1999

7   Last J. *A dictionary of epidemiology. (3rd ed.)* New York: Oxford University Press, 1995

8   Cryer C, Jarvis S, Edwards P *et al.* 'Our Healthier Nation' indicator for unintentional injuries - we can do better. *European Journal of Consumer Safety* 1999;6:183-91

9   Walsh S, Jarvis S. Measuring the frequency of "severe" accidental injury in childhood. *Journal of Epidemiology and Community Health* 1992;46:26-32

10   Jarvis S, Towner E, Walsh S. Accidents. In: Botting B, ed. *The health of our children.* Decennial Supplement OPCS DS No:11. Vol. 95-112. London: HMSO, 1995

11   DiGuiseppi C, Roberts I, Li L. Influence of changing travel patterns on child death rates from injury: trend analysis. *BMJ* 1997;314:710

12   Roberts I, Campbell F, Hollis S *et al.* Reducing accident death rates in children and young adults: The contribution of hospital care. *BMJ* 1996;313:1239-41

13   Department of Health. *Public Health Information Strategy Implementation Project 19. Agreeing an accident information structure.* London: DoH, 1996

14   Department of Health. *An organisation with a memory.* London: The Stationery Office, 2000

15   Department of Health. *Building a safer NHS for patients.* London: The Stationery Office, 2001

16   Jarvis S, Lowe P, Avery A *et al.* Children are not goldfish — mark/recapture techniques and their application to injury data. *Injury Prevention* 2000;6:46-50

17   Edwards P, Kerss M, Jarvis S *et al. PHISSCHing for data. How to implement a monitoring system for injury control and prevention before the next millennium.* University of Newcastle upon Tyne, 1998

18   Morrison A, Stone D, Doraiswamy N *et al.* Injury surveillance in an accident and emergency department: A year in the life of CHIRPP. *Archives of Disease in Childhood* 1999;80:533-6

19 Lyons R, Vui Lon S, Heaven M *et al*. Injury surveillance in children — usefulness of a centralised database of accident and emergency attendances. *Injury Prevention* 1995;1:173-6

20 Bonnie R, Fulco C, Liverman C. *Reducing the burden of injury - advancing prevention and treatment*. Institute of Medicine Committee on Injury Prevention and Control. Washington DC: National Academy Press, 1999

21 US Department of Health and Human Services. *Healthy People 2010: Understanding and Improving Health. (2nd ed.)* Washington, DC: US Government Printing Office, 2000

Chapter 5

1 Ward H and Christie N. *Strategic review of research priorities for accidental injury.* 2000 (http://www.doh.gov.uk/research/documents/rd3/accidental_injuries_report.pdf)

2 Ward H and Christie N. *Strategic review of research priorities for accidental injury.* 2000 (http://www.doh.gov.uk/research/documents/rd3/accidental_injuries_report.pdf)

3 Department of Health. *Saving lives: Our healthier nation.* London: The Stationery Office, 1999

4 Ward H and Christie N. *Strategic review of research priorities for accidental injury.* 2000 (http://www.doh.gov.uk/research/documents/rd3/accidental_injuries_report.pdf)

5 Medical Research Council. *Health of the public programme,* 2001 (http://www.mrc.ac.uk/HOP.html)

Chapter 6

1 Department of Health. *Modernising Social Services: Promoting independence, improving protection, raising standards.* London: The Stationery Office, 1998

2 Department of Health. *Working together to safeguard children: A guide to interagency working to safeguard and promote the welfare of children.* London: The Stationery Office, 1999

3 Department of Health. *Saving lives: Our healthier nation.* London: The Stationery Office, 1999

4 Scottish Office. *Towards a healthier Scotland.* London: The Stationery Office, 1999

5 Welsh Office. *Better health, better Wales.* London: The Stationery Office, 1998

6 Hansard. *Response to Parliamentary Question 132109 tabled by John Austin MP,* 24 July 2000

7   Department of the Environment, Transport and the Regions. *Tomorrow's roads: Safer for everyone. The government's road safety strategy and casualty reduction targets for 2010.* London: The Stationery Office, 2000

8   British Medical Association. *Driving impairment through alcohol and other drugs.* London: BMA, 1996

9   British Medical Association. *Road transport and health.* London: BMA, 1997

10 Department of Health. *Saving lives: Our healthier nation.* London: The Stationery Office, 1999

11 Royal Commission on Environmental Pollution 18th Report. *Transport and the environment.* London: The Stationery Office, 1994

12 National Consultative Forum on Housing in Wales. *Framework for a national housing strategy for Wales,* 1999 (http://www.wales.gov.uk/subihousing/content/framework/contents_e.htm)

13 Her Majesty's Inspectorate of Fire Services for Scotland. *Measuring Up: A consultative paper regarding the Fire Service Inspectorate in Scotland.* Edinburgh: The Stationery Office, 1999

14 Women's Unit and Home Office. *Living without fear: An integrated approach to tackling violence against women.* London: The Stationery Office, 1999

15 Department of Environment, Transport and the Regions. *Revitalising health and safety.* London: The Stationery Office, 2000

16 Towner E, Towner J. Study of effective measures in reducing childhood deaths and serious injuries in 29 OECD countries. *A league table of child deaths by injury in rich nations.* Vol. 13-14. Florence, Italy: UNICEF Innocenti Research Centre, 2001

Appendix 1

1   World Health Organization. *Injury: A leading cause of the global burden of disease.* Geneva: WHO, 1999

2   International Committee of the Red Cross. *27th International Conference of the Red Cross and Red Crescent: Plan of action 2000-2003.* Geneva: ICRC/Federation, 2000

3   Towner E, Towner J. Study of effective measures in reducing childhood deaths and serious injuries in 29 OECD countries. *A league table of child deaths by injury in rich nations.* Vol. 13-14. Florence, Italy: UNICEF Innocenti Research Centre, 2001

4   Baker S. The United States experience: Injury in America. In: Pless B and Towner E, eds. Action on Injury. *Injury Prevention* 4(4) Supplement 1998

5   *Injury in America - a continuing public health problem.* Committee on Trauma Research, Commission on Life Sciences, National Research Council and The Institute of Medicine. Washington DC: National Academy Press, 1985

6   Centres for Disease Control National Centre for Injury Prevention and Control (http://www.cdc.gov/ncipc/ncipchm.htm)

7   Centres for Disease Control National Centre for Injury Prevention and Control (http://www.cdc.gov/ncipc/ncipchm.htm)

8   Rice DP, MacKenzie EJ, Jones AS *et al. Cost of Injury in the United States - a report to Congress.* San Francisco: Institute for Health and Aging, University of California, The Injury Prevention Center, Johns Hopkins University, 1989

9   Injury Prevention: Meeting the Challenge. Committee on Injury Prevention and Control. *American Journal of Preventive Medicine,* Suppl Vol 5; 1989

10 Bonnie RJ, Fulco CE, Liverman CT. *Reducing the burden of injury — Advancing Prevention and Treatment.* Committee on Injury Prevention and Control. Washington DC: Institute of Medicine. National Academy Press, 1999

11 Better Health Commission. *Looking forward to better health.* Canberra: Australian Government Publishing Service, 1986

12 Commonwealth Department of Health and Family Services and the Australian Institute for Health and Welfare. *National Health Priority Areas: Injury prevention and control.* Canberra: Australian Government Publishing Service, 1997

13 Department of Health and Aged Care. *Directions in injury prevention, Report 1: Research needs.* Canberra: National Injury Prevention Council, 1999

14 Department of Health and Aged Care. *Directions in injury prevention, Report 2: Injury Prevention Interventions - good buys for the next decade.* Canberra: National Injury Prevention Council, 1999

15 Australia Department of Human Services and Health. *Better health outcomes for Australians.* Canberra: Australian Government Publishing Service, 1994

16 National Health and Medical Research Council. *Paradigm shift - Injury: from problem to solution.* Canberra: NHMRC, 1999

17 Langley JD, McLoughlin E. *A review of research on unintentional injury.* A report to the Medical Research Council of New Zealand. Special Report Series No 10, Auckland NZ: Medical Research Council, 1987

18 The University of Otago Injury Prevention Research Unit (http://www.otago.ac.nz/ipru/about/about.html)

19 John Langley. *Personal communication,* 2000

Index

academic infrastructure 60, 63, 65
Accident Compensation Corporation
  (New Zealand) (ACC) 94-5, 96
accident and emergency departments
  admission rates 49, 53
  children 13
  data systems 52, 56
  US 91
Accident Task Force 72, 80
accidents
  definition 14
    recommendations 82
Acheson report see Independent
  inquiry into inequalities in health
Action on injury 2
Age Concern 79
aims and scope 4-5
airbags 48
alcohol drinking 22, 44
  driving 17, 44
    BMA policy 73
    Saving lives: Our healthier nation
      25
    QALYs 38
anger control 22
Area Child Protection Committees
  (ACPSs) 71
aspirin, child-safe containers 18, 48
Australia 81, 96
  cost of injuries 29, 30
  injury control policy 92-4
  Looking forward to better health
    30-1
  research 68, 93-4
  road traffic accidents
    children 42, 43
    safety programmes 39-40, 93
Austria 41

avoided death 37
AWISS 56

Better health, better Wales 71
bicycling see cycling
British Medical Association
  Action on injury 2
  The BMA guide to living with risk
    1-2, 3
  Growing up in Britain 2-3
  injury policy 1-2, 78
  Living with risk 1-2
  Road transport and health 73
Building Research Establishment 67
  recommendations 84

Canada 42
  cost of injuries 29, 30
cancers
  disability adjusted life years 34
  funding 35, 63
  potential years of life lost 32-3
  years of life disabled 35
cars 9
causes of injuries see under risk
CCTV 22
Centre for Injury Prevention and
  Control (US) 30
charities 78
  funding 35, 63-4
Child Accident Prevention Trust
  (CAPT) 79
Childline 79
children
  BMA view 2-3
  car safety seats 38, 41-2
  costs of treating injuries 29
  exposure to roads 43, 50

recommendations 82
injuries prevention 3, 18-19, 71, 88
mortality from injuries 8, 9, 10, 41, 58, 81
poisoning 16, 41
child-safe drug containers 16, 18, 48, 84
QALYs 38
risk factors 13, 50
CHIRPP 56
co-ordination of policy 70, 79-81
recommendations 85-6
Cochrane database 66
consultants in rehabilitation 15
consumer product safety 37
child-safe aspirin containers 18, 48
injuries 63
UK policy 52, 70, 76
US policy 57, 91
coronary heart disease, see also stroke 63
coroners' reports 54, 57
recommendations 83
cost-effectiveness 42, 70
injury prevention 36-40
rehabilitation 16
research 61
recommendations 84, 85
costs of treating injuries 29
Crash Outcome Data Evaluation System (CODES) 57
Crime and Disorder Act 1998 75
crowd situations 22-3
cycling 9, 50, 53
data collection 51-2, 54
helmets 20, 38
injuries 13
UK policy 43, 73

data collection 25, 47
recommendations 82
systems 51-4
databases 65, 66
death registration 52, 57

Denmark 41
Department of Culture, Media and Sports 77
Department of the Environment 63
Department of Trade and Industry 63
devolution 70
disability 8, 11, 54
recommendations 82
statistics 51
disability adjusted life years (DALYs) 28, 29
Australia 40
UK 32, 34
recommendations 85
drink driving see under alcohol drinking
drowning 13, 60

economic aspects 27-44
Economic and Social Research Council 65
educational approaches 17, 69
elderly see older people
emergency department see accident and emergency departments
enforcement approaches 17, 69
children 18
cost-effectiveness 37
Engineering and Physical Services Research Council 64
Environment and Healthcare Programme 64-5
environmental approaches 17, 69
children 18
epidemiology
see also occurrence of injury rates 49-50
data 61
research process 62, 63
errors 51
European New Care Assessment Programme (EURO-NCAP) 89
European Union (EU) 58, 76, 88-9
external cause coding 57

falls
    older people 13-14, 47-8
        injury prevention 20-1, 42
    recommendations 84
family therapy 22
Fire Research Station 67
    recommendations 84
fires
    see also smoke alarms 44
    children 13, 41
        smoke alarms 18-19, 42
    research 63
    statistics 49
    UK policy 74-5
football 23
France 19
funding of research 32, 59, 65

general practice
    consultations 11
    injuries burden 10
Germany 42
Glasgow, CHIRPP 56
Growing up in Britain: Ensuring a
    healthy future for our children 2-3
gun control 44

head injuries 16, 53, 64
Health action zones 25
Health Development Agency 67
health impact assessment 85
Health improvement programmes 26
health inequalities 4
    injury prevention 23-4
    recommendations 84
health promotion 67, 78
Health of the Public 64
Health Public Service Agreement 72
Health and Safety Commission (HSC)
    3
Health and Safety Executive (HSE)
    crowd guidance 22-3
    research programme 63
    UK policy 77

work accident rates 49, 52
Health and Safety Laboratory 67
    recommendations 84
health surveillance 45-6
Health Survey for England (HsurvE)
    52, 53
Healthy People 2010 (US) 58
Help the Aged 79
home injuries 61
    children 13
    UK policy 59, 74
Home and Leisure Accident
    Surveillance System (HASS/LASS)
    52, 53, 53-4, 54
    EU 88-9
    UK policy 76
Home Office 63
homicide 9
hospital admission rates 11, 49
    hospital episode data (HES) 52, 53,
        54
    older people 14
housing
    UK policy 73
    Wales 74, 80

Independent inquiry into inequalities
    in health 23-4
injuries
    definitions 4, 49
        recommendations 82
    epidemiology 7, 8
    mortality 8-9
        social class 10
    severity 49, 57
        recommendations 83
Injury: A leading cause of the global
    burden of disease 87-8
Injury in America 30
injury data systems 51-4
injury hazards 50
injury prevention 14-26
    BMA view 2
    children 18-19

cost-effectiveness 36-40
health inequalities 23-4
implementation 40-2
policy structures 70
research 59
tertiary prevention 15-16
UK spending 36
Injury prevention and control 92
Injury Prevention Programme (EU) 58
injury surveillance 45-58
  characteristics 47-8
  definition 46
  recommendations 81-3
Institute of Child Health 78
intentional injuries
  child poisoning 16
  children 10
  injury prevention 21-2
  mortality, social class 10
  UK policy 71, 75, 80
  recommendations 84
International Classification of Diseases
  (ICD) 57
  recommendations 83
International Classification of External
  Causes of Injuries (ICECI) 57
International Collaborative Effort on
  Injury Statistics 58
international injury surveillance 58
International Labour Organization
  (ILO) 88
International Road Research
  Documentation (IRRD) 66
internet 68
ischaemic heart disease
  disability adjusted life years UK 34
  potential years of life lost in UK 32-3
  years of life disabled 35

Joint Futures Group 71
journals 65

Living with risk 1-2
Living without fear 75

long-term consequences of injuries see
  under disability
Looking forward to better health 30-1

marginal costs 41
Measuring up 75
Medical Research Council(MRC) 35, 64
Medline database 66
Melbourne declaration 79
mental health 21
minor injuries 11, 67
mistakes see under errors
Modernising social services 71
monitoring 66
morbidity see under disability
mortality
  injuries 8-9
    children 8, 9, 10, 41, 58, 81
    social class 10
  rate reductions 50-1
  road traffic accidents 88
motorcycle helmets 20
multi-disciplinary research 65
  recommendations 84

National Association of Citizens Advice
  Bureaux 76
National Center for Health Statistics
  (US) 57
National Center for Injury Prevention
  (US) 58, 90, 91, 96
National Community Fire Safety
  Centre 74
National Electronic Surveillance
  System (NEISS) (US) 57, 91, 92
National Highway Traffic Safety
  Administration (US) 57, 91
National Injury Surveillance Unit
  (Australia) 93, 96
National Patient Safety Agency 51
National Research Register (NRR) 64,
  66, 66-7
National service framework for mental
  health services in England 21, 25

National service frameworks for older people 25
National Society for the Prevention of Cruelty to Children (NSPCC) 78-9
near misses see under errors
Netherlands
    cost of injuries 29, 30
    road traffic accidents 19, 41
New Zealand 81, 96
    cost of injuries 29
    injury control policy 94-5
    research 31
Newcastle, PHISSCH 55
NHS Common Services Agency 7
NHS Direct 53
non-fatal injuries 10-11, 50
Northern Ireland 71, 72
    mortality from injuries 8-9
Norway 42

occupational health 3
    accidents 49, 52, 77-8
    EU 88
    recommendations 85
occurrence of injury rates, see also epidemiology 49-50
Office of Fair Trading 76
Office for National Statistics 78
Official Group on Violence against Women 75
older people
    falls 13-14, 47-8
    incidence of injuries 8
    injury prevention 20-1
    risk factors 13-14, 21
    road exposure 43
Our healthier nation 2
ownership of injury problem 60, 63

parenting skills 22
Parliamentary All-party Advisory Committee on Transport Safety (PACTS) 78
pedestrian injuries

see also road traffic accidents 43, 50
    children 19
    data collection 51-2
PHISSCH 55
Play Safety Forum 77
poisoning 60
    child-safe drug containers 16, 18, 48
        recommendations 84
    children 13
police 75
post-traumatic stress disorders 11
potential years of life lost (PYLL) 28
    UK 32-3
    US 31
poverty and health see under health inequalities
primary care groups 14, 26
primary prevention 16, 62
Psychinfo database 66

quality adjusted life years (QALYs) 37-9

recommendations 81-6
Red Cross 88
Reducing the burden of injury 92
regional NHS Executive offices 67
register of research 66, 68
rehabilitation 15-16, 25, 60, 64
reporting of injuries, diseases and dangerous occurrences (RIDDOR) 52
research 30-6, 59-68
    Australia 93-4
    dissemination 67-8
    monitoring 66-7
    process 62
    UK funding 32, 59, 65
    US 91
    recommendations 83
risk
    exposure to 50
    factors 12-14, 20
    nature of 1-2

research process 62
road safety
    see also transport safety
    UK policy 73, 80
road traffic accidents
    see also pedestrian injuries
    airbags 48
    BMA policy 73
    children 13, 41, 43
    cost-effectiveness 39
    data collection 49, 52, 53
    EU 89
    injury surveillance 48, 50
    mortality 88
    research 59, 63
    risks 12
    Saving lives: Our healthier nation
        25, 73
    Scotland 76-7
    seat belts 24, 50, 84
    UK policy 72-4
    young people 13, 20
    recommendations 83
Road transport and health 73
Royal Commission on Environmental
    Pollution 73
Royal Society for the Prevention of
    Accidents (RoSPA) 79
rural injuries 12, 60

Saving lives: Our healthier nation 24-
    5, 48, 71, 73
Scotland 70, 72
    education 76-7
    fire safety 74-5
    mortality from injuries 8-9
seat belts 24, 50
    recommendations 84
secondary prevention 16, 62
severity of injuries 49, 57
    recommendations 83
smoke alarms
    see also fires 18-19, 23, 42
    QALYs 38

Saving lives: Our healthier nation 25
    recommendations 82, 84
smoking 42
social class 10
Social Research Council 65
speed limits 19
    recommendations 84
spinal injuries 64
sports injuries 12, 53, 60, 61
    UK policy 77
    recommendations 83
standard gamble methods 37
Statistics Commission 78
STATS19 data 52, 53, 54
    recommendations 83
stroke
    see also coronary heart disease
    disability adjusted life years 34
    potential years of life lost 32-3
    years of life disabled 35
suicide 4
    injury prevention 21
    mortality 9
Sure start 77
survival rates 51
Sweden 41, 42, 43
swimming pools 41

tariff values 39-40
tertiary prevention 15-16
    research process 62
time trade-off methods 37
Tomorrow's roads: Safer for everyone
    72
Towards a healthier Scotland 71
Trading standards officers 76
Transport Research Laboratory 67, 78
    recommendations 84
transport safety, see also road safety 78
Trauma Audit and Research Network
    (TARN) 52, 53, 53-4, 54
trauma services 15

undetermined injuries 10

UNICEF 88
unintentional injuries
  child-safe drug containers 13, 18
    recommendations 84
  children 10, 13, 55
  mortality 9
    social class 10
  prevention methods 17
  research
    priorities 59-60
    process 62
    register 66
  UK policy 71, 71-2, 80
  young people 13
United Nations 79
United States 81
  cost of injuries 29, 30
  Injury in America 30
  injury control policy 90-2
  Injury prevention and control 92
  injury surveillance system 57, 91, 92
  International Collaborative Effort on
    Injury Statistics 58
  motor cycle helmets 20
  National Center for Injury
    Prevention 58, 90
  potential years of life lost 31
  Reducing the burden of injury 92
  research 68, 91
  road traffic accidents 91
  smoke alarms 18, 42
  water heaters 18

window guards 18
urban safety programme 39

violence
  injury prevention 21-2
  women 75
visual analogue methods 37

Wales 71, 72, 74
  AWISS 56
  housing policy 74, 80
  mortality from injuries 8-9
water heaters 18
Wellcome Trust 64
window guards 18, 42
women 75, 80
work 3
World Bank 79
World Conference on Injury
  Prevention and Control 79
World Health Assembly 79
World Health Organization (WHO) 7, 79
  The global burden of disease 29
  Injury: A leading cause of the
    burden of disease 87
  research spending 31-2

years of life disabled (YLD) 28
  UK 34, 35
young people
  injury prevention 20
  risk factors 13